Stefan Ball is a consultant at the Dr Edward Bach Centre, which is the centre founded by Dr Bach to continue his work with flower essences. He is also a director of the Dr Edward Bach Foundation, the worldwide education and registration organisation for Bach practitioners. He is the author of several books, including *The Bach Remedies Workbook* and *Bach Flower Remedies for Men*.

bloom

*Using flower essences for personal development
and spiritual growth*

Stefan Ball

Vermilion
LONDON

1 3 5 7 9 10 8 6 4 2

First published in 2006 by Vermilion,
an imprint of Ebury Publishing, Random House,
20 Vauxhall Bridge Road, London SW1V 2SA

Random House Australia (Pty) Limited
20 Alfred Street, Milsons Point, Sydney,
New South Wales 2061, Australia

Random House New Zealand Limited
18 Poland Road, Glenfield,
Auckland 10, New Zealand

Random House South Africa (Pty) Limited
Isle of Houghton, Corner Boundary Road & Carse O'Gowrie,
Houghton 2198, South Africa

The Random House Group Limited Reg. No. 954009

Papers used by Vermilion are natural, recyclable products made from wood grown
in sustainable forests.

Printed and bound in Great Britain by Mackays of Chatham Ltd, Chatham, Kent

A CIP catalogue record for this book
is available from the British Library

ISBN 009190678-4

✿ Contents

Growth is the only evidence of life.

Cardinal Newman, *Apologia pro Vita Sua*

emotion / <u>n.</u> [f. L *emovere*, f. E- + *movere* move.]
2 A migration; a change of position.

The New Shorter Oxford English Dictionary,
volume 1, A–M

❀ introduction

a legend

Long ago in China a young man of fashion called Keu Tze Tung offended the emperor. In fear of his life Tung fled the city and took refuge in a hidden valley. There he learned a sacred message, which he painted onto the petals of pure flowers. He watched the dew that formed on the petals and drank it as it dripped. The dew contained the power of the sacred text. It made him immortal.

This book is about a discovery made by a doctor from Birmingham in the English West Midlands. He too fled a city – London – and took refuge in the country. He too found a special power in the dew that forms on flowers. And while the messages in each flower didn't make him immortal …

practical, down to earth, real

'Yes, it's all very interesting, but I haven't got time for it. I've got a lot to do and I just want to get on with it.'

I was talking to a middle-aged lady, an unwilling visitor to the Bach Centre. Her elderly mother had persuaded her to turn off the London to Oxford road and visit the small Victorian cottage that was Dr Edward Bach's home up until his death in 1936. I admit that I couldn't understand her objection. 'Getting on with it' is exactly what Bach's work is all about.

Bach was a well-known bacteriologist, pathologist and homoeopath whose career included spells at University College Hospital and the London Homoeopathic Hospital as well as a successful Harley Street practice. His orthodox research received great acclaim but left him unsatisfied, and in 1928 he began to experiment with medicines made from flowers.

Bach had always been more interested in the people suffering disease than in the diseases themselves, a fact that set him apart from the mainstream medicine of his time. He was looking for a way to treat the emotional imbalances that were in his view the underlying cause of illness. He found an affinity between emotional states and the energy in certain flowering plants and trees. He made thirty-eight remedies from these plants, each one aimed at a particular mood or characteristic.

The remedies worked by encouraging latent qualities in people so as to drive out negative thoughts and behaviour. They produced profound effects in such a gentle way that mothers could give them without fear to their new-born babies. They didn't alter the personality or bring instant nirvana. Instead they brought people gently back to themselves so they could go on learning from their lives. Well-balanced people got better physically as their bodies returned to their normal and natural state of health. And the most remarkable thing about the remedies was their simplicity. The thirty-eight formed a complete system. People could mix them together like primary colours so as to match every shade of human emotion. Because there were so few remedies, with clear indications for each one, the system fell within the reach of anyone who took the trouble to learn it.

The simple and profound system Bach discovered continues today as it was then, and is more popular than ever before. The Dr Edward Bach Foundation registers practitioners in forty-one different countries. Several manufacturers make the thirty-eight essences, which come ready-to-use in little glass bottles with droppers in the caps, and the longest-established and best-known manufacturer exports to nearly seventy countries around the world. Pharmacies, health food shops, even supermarkets stock them alongside the cough medicines and vitamin pills. The British royal family is said to use them. So do pop stars and models and actors, and students and housewives and lawyers and doctors and nurses and midwives and businessmen and -women. Hardly a day goes by without some reference to them in print or on TV or radio. Almost every feature on stress, relationship breakdown or the contents of famous people's pockets and handbags includes one or two flower essences as a matter of course.

Popularisation at this level stresses the simple more than the profound, particularly when tight deadlines force magazine writers to produce copy with no time for research or understanding. Over the years I have taken many calls from harassed journalists who have only just heard of flower essences but still need to produce a thousand words within a few hours. Soundbites and clichés rule the media – 'give me something quick and easy to understand' – and like everyone else involved in the essences I have done my share of soundbiting and have helped string together two-minute introductions and quotable quips on demand. The cumulative effect of this has been to promote a few easy-to-understand essences at the expense of the whole system. In particular the ready-prepared combination best known under the trade name Rescue™ Remedy has become something of a media icon. As the name implies, Bach put Rescue™ Remedy together as a quick fix for use in crises. Journalists with a deadline and no time love it. Its name says what it is for. It has immediate grab and appeal in a way that the single remedies, all named after flowers, don't. People who claim never to have heard of Bach still have a bottle of Rescue™ Remedy on their desk. It is complementary medicine's answer to the Band-Aid™, something we all use without stopping to ask too many questions.

The success of Rescue™ Remedy is marvellous, but it is also limiting. Many of its fans never move beyond it. It's as if their sole knowledge of allopathic (orthodox) medicine began and ended with the sticking plaster.

the meaning of advanced

This is a great shame. The process of matching essences to the way we feel can do more than patch us up and get us through today's crisis. If we turn to the full system we can discover whole new layers to our personalities and whole new areas of potential growth. We can change our lives. *Bloom* aims to help us use flower essences in this more advanced way – and by 'advanced' I mean deeper, fuller, more profound.

Simplicity and profundity don't have to oppose each other. 'Advanced' doesn't mean moving away from the simple 'kitchen cabinet' approach that Bach took or getting bogged down in esoteric or pseudo-scientific mumbo-jumbo. Instead this book is about simplicity as a frame of mind, one that helps us take an active part in our own spiritual and emotional evolution, and one that fits in with whatever spiritual beliefs we espouse. I will argue that the simplest approach to using flower essences has the most profound spiritual effects. It helps us realise our potential and advance along our life's path. It helps us rediscover our relationship with the world and with life itself. And the deep, life-changing, profound, *advanced* use of these remedies can start any day that we decide to take a single flower for a single pressing problem.

'I don't look on the remedies as something to be used only when ill,' says Angela Day, a practitioner and teacher in the south-east of England. 'I see them as something to be used in a very natural way just as I use food and drink. My set of remedies sits on my kitchen dresser, readily and easily available, so I can take them as and when I feel the need. I see them as something that keeps me together and allows me to be more myself.'

It is as simple as that.

using this book

Reading is always a linear journey. We read books from cover to cover; the questions posed in the introduction are answered in the conclusion. Life is different. The route through life is never straight. It doubles back on itself and is full of twists and turns. We can't work through life – or through a list of flower essences – in any one order and expect to come out the other side. Nor can we expect to deal with each part of life – or each essence – once and once only. Life will bring us back to where we started several times. When we think we are closest to its centre we may be furthest away, and we may be closest to our heart when we think we are at the outer limits of our journey.

Aware of this, many essence users think of the flowers and their related emotional qualities as friends rather than medicines to be taken and discarded. Friends revisit us and we revisit them. They help us over and over again. The longer we know them the more sides to them we see. Sometimes one particular friend will be enough to pick us up when we are down. Sometimes we need several, one after the other, or all at once. 'There is more than one friend in the remedies,' says Noëlle Mogridge, who has been using the thirty-eight essences for nearly forty years. 'I've smiled at my Crab Apple self, slowed down with Impatiens, fortified myself with Hornbeam on the slow days when I just couldn't get around to doing anything. I have chosen Scleranthus when I've had choices to make, gratefully accepted White Chestnut in times of turmoil, protected myself with Walnut, and wearily reached for the Olive when I've busied myself to bits.' Another user, Richard, would agree. 'They have been like a very special friend to me,' he says, 'always there when needed, always giving of their best when I call on them, bringing a higher and deeper vibration into my life – a gift from nature, aiding my clarity and insight by allowing me to be more centred in the midst of my process, a constant reminder and inspiration to explore myself.'

In the task of exploring ourselves we can choose where to begin, and pick out a path, or just begin and see where the path takes us. We must always have a choice, and with this in mind I have provided three main paths through this book.

❀ *If you are new to flower essences but already involved in personal growth* read chapters i to vii. These deal with Bach's seven essence groups and tell you when to take each flower and what it will do for you. Chapter i starts on page 13.

❀ *If you know the essences quite well but are only starting to think about personal growth* read chapters 1 to 7. They show how the thirty-eight remedies relate to downshifting, peak experiences and religious and philosophical belief. I have also used this space to make a political argument about how we should best use Bach's flower essences. Chapter 1 starts on page 1.

❀ *If you want to take time to think about both subjects* just keep reading from here. This is the simplest way to read any book, and in *this* book simplicity is always its own recommendation.

Which path we walk depends on what we want to do and where we are coming from. All three paths in *Bloom* are linear — such is the restriction of the form — but I have tried to make each of them open out into the much wider and more ornate path of life itself. If I have managed to do this it is thanks to the many people like Angela, Noëlle and Richard who have shared their experiences and thoughts with me. If I have failed the fault is my own.

> Having access to the remedies is a bit like having a friend or neighbour you know you can rely on in times of need – not interfering in any way, but simply there for you.
> – Caroline Hedicker

❀ acknowledgements

I have listed all the books I have read, consulted and plundered at the back of the book, but I wanted to mark out a few special debts.

In writing about Bach's life I have followed Nora Weeks's biography, still the only reliable published source. Weeks knew Bach for many years, and was with him throughout the period during which the remedies were discovered. People often assume that they were lovers, but there is no evidence this was true. Long after his death she still referred to him as 'the doctor', which suggests their intimacy remained that of close colleagues and friends.

I first read Colin Wilson's *The Outsider* more than twenty years ago. I lent it to my friends and we spent many enjoyable nights getting drunk and arguing about it. In those days I accepted the analysis but not the conclusions. The book's main and most lasting influence was to persuade me to read or re-read Nietzsche, Camus, Sartre, Eliot, Dostoyevsky, Kafka, Hemingway, Hesse and others. I used *The Outsider* like the contents page of a course in philosophy and fiction. Even today I get a thrill out of turning up in a second-hand bookshop some text that Wilson mentioned in passing. In preparing to write this book I re-read *The Outsider* and re-read in turn many of the books it mentions. To my surprise I now accept (some of) Wilson's conclusions more than (some of) his analysis, but the book is still important to me and I'm grateful for it.

Some influences on this book have been the result of happy coincidence (or synchronicity if you prefer). When I was puzzling over the presentation of Walnut, for example, I happened to hear a radio announcer mention Chabrier's encounter with Wagner's music. A couple of paragraphs fell into place. The same thing happened when I was struggling to remember scenes and themes from the film

Koyaanisqatsi. Picking up a TV listings magazine, there it was in the film guide, being broadcast for the first time in ten or more years.

Lynn Macwhinnie and Judy Howard both read the text in draft and made helpful and sometimes challenging suggestions, as did my editor at Vermilion, Sue Lascelles. Many others have helped towards this book in one way or another – mostly by providing the personal testimonies referred to throughout the text. Some are named in the text, some appear under pseudonyms. In any case I wanted to thank in particular Andrée Samuel, Nicola Hanefeld, Katya Cozic, Theresa McInnes, Christine Newman, Cath Harper, Karen Briscombe, Una McRory, Lynn Hinton, Rosemary Barry, Hermia Brockway, Elaine Copeland, Nobuko Asanuma, Di Bradley, Diana Antonaroli, Helen Kent, Sandra-Elizabeth Ross, Helga Braun, Jeff Chambers, Alison Evans, Aileen Falconer, Cynthia Prior, Andrea Williams, Linda Beckenham, Gillian Smith, Angela Day, Tracey Deacon, Ian McPherson, John Logan, Alice Walkingshaw, Sheila Bennett, Helen Lawton, Angela Davies, Beth Darrall, Julie Lloyd-Jenkins, Catherine Gurnet, Miki Hayashi, Jackie Lowy, Jill Woods, Elaine Arthey, Michael Hillier, Hilary Leigh, Charles Callis, Alison Lock, David Brandon, Florence Salooja, Maureen Murphy, Susanne McAllister, Kate Anderson, Yurina Shiraishi, Evelyn Munro, Liz Bailey, Flor Tavor, Caroline Windsor, Susan Rigg, Sylvia Spence, Katrina Mountfort, Alison Murphy, Debbie Henderson, Maggie Evans, Claire Hingley, Claire Bickerton, Anna Richardson, Margaret Blackman, Alison Hudd, Lynne Crescenzo, Deirdre Barron, Judy Beveridge, Pamela Higginson, Aneeta Chakravarty, Martine Eyre, Elaine Abel, Frances O'Sullivan, Stuart Guffogg, Valerie Miller, Noëlle Mogridge, Julia Barker, Janice Cracknell, Janet Duffill, Susan Robinson, Lynn Hall, Elaine More, Caroline Hedicker, Avril Harvey, Christine Racquez, Pamela Wells, Lynne Langley, Sylvia Rymer-Lawes, Linda Lewcock, Rixt Spierings, Andrea Allardyce, Katya Cozic and Christine Philp.

As usual I owe several nods of gratitude to my family and to everybody at the Bach Centre. Thank you, thank you, thank you.

❀ three notes on names and gender

For many years the words 'Bach' and 'Bach Flower Remedies' were registered trade marks used first by the Bach Centre and then by A. Nelson & Co to identify remedies containing mother tinctures made at the Bach Centre. Outside the UK 'Bach', 'Bach Flower Remedies' and 'Bach Flower Essences' continue to be trade marks or registered trade marks and continue to have that meaning, but following a decision by the UK High Court in 1998 the words 'Bach' and 'Bach Flower Remedies' are no longer registered trade marks within the UK. Because I am writing in the UK I have followed the current UK convention and have written 'Bach flower remedies' or 'Bach remedies' using the lower case. This should not be seen as invalidating or failing to acknowledge any trade marks in use anywhere in the world.

The usual meaning of the word 'remedies' suggests that we need to have something medically wrong with us before we can start to take them. For this reason, and given that this book is about personal development rather than health as such, I wanted to move away from using the word 'remedies' as the sole synonym for Bach's thirty-eight preparations. Nevertheless, 'remedies' was one of Bach's own preferred terms and was not to be discarded lightly. After much thought I kept it, then, but also used 'essences' and 'flowers' where this felt appropriate, encouraged by the fact that both these descriptors are widely used outside the UK in association with Bach's discoveries. I don't pretend that either is more exact than 'remedies'. Indeed both are open to challenge. In every other branch of medicine and chemistry a plant essence is an extremely concentrated extract; Bach flower 'essences' are highly dilute. And one of the 'flowers' (Rock Water) is not made with a plant at all.

On the subject of tricky conventions, I have once again had to grasp the nettle of the personal pronoun problem. I decided always to use 'she' when talking about potential positive and negative remedy archetypes as if they were real individuals. To balance this I mainly use 'he' when talking about mere mortals – the man in the street or on the Clapham omnibus or in the laboratory. I intend offence neither to mortal women nor archetypal males, and hope both will forgive me my pedantic refusal to write 'they', 'them' and 'their' when I mean one person.

Now what is the flower for that...?

1 ❀ life out of balance

things

'It's the economy, stupid!'

When Bill Clinton ran for the US presidency in 1992 his campaign manager hung this sign at the back of his press conferences to remind the candidate not to stray from the most important topic. Politicians are especially wedded to the idea that increasing material wealth is our overriding concern. Material wealth seems easy to measure, weigh and compare. Government and opposition alike can gesture towards national product and rates of taxation and inflation as self-evident reasons for the electorate to be content or discontent. We can see and feel our happiness when we look at the things we have accumulated, the money in the bank, the size of our house and the power of our car. Nobody need make further analysis.

Unfortunately this is a fallacy, as the social psychologist David Myers shows in *The Pursuit of Happiness*, a review of research into what makes people happy. In poor countries more things do indeed bring more contentment. But beyond a certain point the law of diminishing returns kicks in, until in the rich countries we barely notice our fluctuating wealth. More things have little effect and the curve of happiness levels off. In Myers's words, whatever the measure we use 'our becoming better-off over the last thirty years has not been accompanied by one iota of increased happiness and life satisfaction.' So it's not the economy, stupid, and if we think beyond the slogan it should be obvious. We live the same number of hours in a day as our most remote ancestors. As the things pile up the hours fill until we have more things than time. How many CDs do we own that we haven't played in the last year? How many books on our shelves have never been read? How many ornaments and pictures do we never look at or take pleasure from? Hardly surprising that a few things more or less barely register when we think about happiness.

We are addicted to consumerism, as junkies are to heroin and drinkers are to booze. Feeling something is missing from our lives, we go into retail therapy and buy more. And buying more things means earning more money to pay for them. 'A depressing number of Americans believe,' writes Lewis Lapham, 'that if only they had twice as much, they would inherit the estate of happiness promised them in the Declaration of Independence. The man who receives $15,000 a year is sure that he could relieve his sorrow if he had only $30,000 a year; the man with $1 million a year knows that all would be well if he had $2 million a year.' According to a poll published in the USA in 1995 by the Merck Family Fund twenty-seven per cent of people earning more than $100,000 a year said they could not afford to buy everything they needed. Somebody once asked John D. Rockefeller what was enough. 'Just one more,' he said.

Rockefeller was wrong. Too many things can actually make our lives worse. Lottery winners often feel less happy than before because their sudden wealth cuts them off from the very things that gave their lives structure and meaning: making their own entertainment, cooking, taking care of children, going to work, meeting friends who understand the same problems. They realise too late that what they needed was not money but a reason to get out of bed in the morning. Perhaps it's fortunate then that money makes work and can become a full-time and stressful occupation, full of new worries. Have we invested it well enough? What if we lose it? What if the stock market falls? Do we have enough insurance to replace everything if there is a fire? What if our accountant steals from us? How much do we stand to lose if we get divorced?

sacrifices

Economic wealth and material prosperity involve sacrifice. They cost time and energy that we could have used in other ways. Take parent–child relationships as an example. Many parents believe they need two incomes in order to give themselves and their children the standard of living to which they aspire. The pursuit of success at work leads parents to work longer hours so that contact time with children is reduced. According to research published in 2000, sixty per cent of British parents no longer have time to read a bedtime story to their children. This compares to the mid-1970s when three-quarters of all children were read to by Mum or Dad. In those days a third of children enjoyed a story every night; now this has halved to just sixteen per cent. And the most common complaint made by children about their parents' reading to them was that their fathers fell asleep halfway through the story. The position is the same in the US: the current generation of American parents spends forty per cent less time with its children than their parents did with them. Saying 'yes' to more work and more money and more things means saying 'no' to time with the kids, and to many other basic human pleasures: friends, nature, meditation, leisure, time to think and read.

It has often been pointed out that nobody ever died wishing to have spent more time in the office, but have we listened? How sure are we that we will not one day face the conclusion that Henry David Thoreau made up his mind to avoid when he went to walk and live in the woods? 'I wished to live deliberately,' he wrote in *Walden*, 'to confront all of the essential facts of life, and see if I could learn what it had to teach, and not, when I came to die, to discover that I had not lived.'

koyaanisqatsi

The Hopi tribe in North America have a word for our madness: *koyaanisqatsi*. It means 'crazy life', 'disintegrating life' or 'life in turmoil'.

But my favourite translation, which has stayed in my mind long after I saw the film of the same title in the mid-1980s, is 'life out of balance'.

The film opens with a slow shot of a rock painting in a womb-like desert cave. We get the impression of peace and great age — all is still and quiet, and the paintings, and by extension human life, seem as old and natural as the cave itself. The focus moves outside to the desert, the Grand Canyon, mountains. Cloud formations and the movement of sun and shadow across the landscape emphasise the natural rhythms of life. Then, all at once, we are flying over vast fields of monoculture as we leave natural life behind and enter the teeming world of mechanisation and modern humanity.

The stillness and natural rhythms of nature and the cave paintings have gone. Vast globular power stations and gleaming metal towers rise out of polluted landscapes like monstrous boils. Sunbathers and trash and patches of artificial colour litter the beaches. Soon we are in the city and the pace picks up. Citizens move at lightning speed and in great masses, stepping on and off escalators and feeding through stations and streets. The city has a monstrous life of its own, while the humans inside it are either automata, reacting to the lights and signals around without thought, or products, fed through tubes and channels like sausage meat. There is no rest in a world where even leisure time is frenetic. People bowling, eating, watching a film are all constantly in motion, twitching, shifting about. At night figures in lighted apartments move without cease, their wanderings traced by the turning on and off of the lights. In the sky, ignored, the ancient moon drifts past until we lose sight of it behind a skyscraper.

Towards the end of the film the camera picks faces out of the crowd. A worker in a power station smokes a cigarette. A man shaves himself in a crowded street, unaware of the swarms breaking to each side of him like water around a rock. A young couple peer suspiciously from side to side. An old man stands lost, hopeless and alone in the crowd. Far from being Nietzschean supermen enjoying unlimited power, the inhabitants of the glittering web are helpless and alone. Alienated as much from each other as from the natural world, they have no connection with the crowd or with the city. In the final frames they become ghosts, barely visible against the hard outlines of their installations.

Koyaanisqatsi illustrates some fundamental truths. Its avowed intent, explained in the last frames when the dictionary definitions of the title appear on the screen, is to show what a crazy life, a life out of balance, looks and feels like. It succeeds in creating useful reference points. Four of them in particular stand out.

- ❄ **Lack of control.** People mill about in cities built for giants. They lack inner life and self-determination. They are swept along by their material creations and seem unable to control their environment or their lives.
- ❄ **Lack of stillness.** People rush everywhere. On the few occasions when they stop moving they seem bored and ill at ease.
- ❄ **Loneliness.** People seem isolated and unable to make contact with the crowds around them. They are anxious, disturbed and disconnected.
- ❄ **Disrespect for nature.** The city feeds off nature's raw materials yet ignores natural rhythms. Consumption is an end in itself. Pollution and humanity's weapons threaten to destroy the whole planet.

To put it another way, a life out of balance is one in which we abandon the right to choose our own path, place doing above being – 'we spend more and more time as a *human doing* and less and less as a *human being*,' writes psychologist Robert Holden – and lose our connections to others and to the wider universe. These themes will recur in this book over and over, for any attempt at a balanced life has to come to terms in one way or another with every one of them.

pleasure

It was a cold day in October. I lived in London and I was out of work. I spent the morning and early afternoon sitting by a one-bar electric fire reading a library copy of Mervyn Peake's *Gormenghast*. In the afternoon I broke off from reading and went to the park. There I ran around the athletics track for nearly an hour. It began to get dark. I jogged home, changed and sat back in front of the fire. I remember the delight of picking up the book again so as to find out what would happen to Steerpike.

Nowadays one of my favourite places is Wittenham Clumps in Oxfordshire, a few miles from where I live. The clumps are two rounded hills with woods and fields behind falling down to the Thames. The clump on the left has a small fenced-off wood at the top – the trustees protect the wood because it is part of a wildlife reserve. Up by the fence is where you find the kite-flyers and lovers of long-distance views. Off on the right is the second clump, an Iron Age and later Roman hill fort. This too has a beech wood on top, though this one is not fenced and you can walk through it. One of the trees, long dead now, is known locally as the Poem Tree because a Victorian gentleman carved a long poem into its bark. As the tree grew the words and letters ballooned out into strange shapes, making them hard to read. A pillar nearby reproduces it for those who struggle to read the original. Behind the hill fort tracks lead around and down into a pine wood before joining up with the main path from the first hill and curving away to Day's Lock and the small bridge over the Thames where Winnie-the-Pooh played pooh sticks.

Here is another memory. (Please forgive the self-indulgence.) I was visiting a girlfriend in France, near to the Swiss border. It was winter. My girlfriend's brother and his friend were visiting the house as well, and were enthusiastic skiers. It was apparently a perfect day for skiing. After some discussion in French – which at the time I could barely follow – they decided to go to the mountains and take me with them. I had never been skiing before and the easy route seemed to be to go along and give it a try. But skiing and I parted company that day and will never again be friends. Everything cost a lot of money at a time when I didn't have any: hire of boots, ski pass, lift pass, food, drink. The ski centre was wet, crowded and dirty, full of souvenir shops and the worst kind of tourist kitsch. I didn't have the right clothes and consequently I froze. Skiing itself was much harder than it looked. By a combination of luck and misdirected effort I eventually ended up a long way downhill of the ski centre, and away from the lifts. I remember the grim struggle up the mountain to get back to the top. Above all I remember the penetrating cold and the desperate wish to be anywhere else.

OK, I'm a wimp. I could have said 'no', and having said 'yes' I should have tried harder to enjoy the experience. In retrospect I can think of a number of essences that would have helped me be less of a wet blanket. And millions of people love skiing and go as often as they can. I'm not attacking skiing or people who like skiing, or crowds or people who like crowds – or people who like souvenir shops. I'm just making two points.

- ❀ *First*, that there is great and lasting pleasure in the small things in life.
- ❀ *Second*, that expensive things that involve a lot of consumption – aeroplane flights, special equipment, expensive food and drink – are often neither enjoyable nor rewarding nor satisfying.

These points need making because so much of the modern world wants to tell us that expensive and wasteful is upbeat and fun, and cheap and quiet is downbeat and boring. The media is especially to blame. Take a look at television advertising, and at the programmes it interrupts. Take a look at children's TV in particular. Thirty years ago we had a mix of programmes in the UK. The frantic comedy of *Crackerjack* and *Batman* gave way to gentle and reflective shows like *Animal Magic* and *Tales of the Riverbank*. In *Jackanory* somebody sat on a chair and told a tale, carrying on a tradition of oral storytelling that stretches back hundreds of thousands of years into prehistory. In contrast, today's children's TV seems based on the belief that the only way to get a child's attention is to shout and do everything at ninety miles an hour. And all the programmes, from the cartoons up, promote something, whether it's someone's new CD or video, a new game or toy, action figures, hairstyles, entry to theme parks or the latest clothes.

We and our children are overwhelmed by demands, opportunities, pressures and expectations. There is too much going on, so many things and activities competing for our time, so many fashions to follow and tribes to join. The result, I believe, is that we are pressured into consumption instead of taking time to think about what we really want to be. As a society, as a race, we are becoming like me going on my skiing trip: whisked along by the enthusiasms of others, out of our own control, unable to say 'no' or stand still through lack of time and comprehension. And in our helter-skelter slide through life we only rarely stop and think about how happy we really are.

needs

In 1962 the psychologist Abraham Maslow set out his ideas about human needs in a book called *Towards a Psychology of Being*. According to Maslow, needs can be understood as a hierarchy, something like a pyramid. We start at the bottom of the pyramid and move up through the levels as our circumstances improve. At the bottom Maslow put the fundamentals such as food to feed us, shelter from the elements and air to breathe. These needs are basic because we die if we can't meet them. If we have a problem at this level – say, for example, we struggle to get enough to eat – we will not be able to think about anything else and so will not move up the hierarchy. But once we *have* satisfied our basic needs our focus moves away to the next level, where we begin to think about safety and comfort, then to our need to find friendship, love and a place in society. And once these needs are met our focus changes again to the need for esteem. We want to be able to respect ourselves and to have the respect of others. We want to feel confident and useful and valuable. At each stage the satisfaction of one set of needs shifts the focus to the next highest storey of the pyramid.

Maslow placed the *self-actualisation* needs at the top of the hierarchy. Self-actualisation includes two complementary components:

❀ *First*, finding one's particular path in life, or self-development.
❀ *Second*, feeling connected to something greater than oneself, or the transcending of self.

The great self-actualisers in history have been religious leaders such as Mohammed, Jesus and Buddha, but we find the same combination in great artists, musicians and poets, political leaders and campaigners of all kinds.

Maslow pointed out that the failure to meet felt needs results in unhappiness and restlessness regardless of the level of the pyramid we have reached. If we fail to find love and affection we will be unhappy, but finding love and affection will not in itself lead to permanent happiness because we will begin to look for respect. Continuing happiness is therefore a process in which we shift the focus up the pyramid and meet successive needs as we get to them. And our natural tendency to move up the hierarchy explains why the consumer culture fails to satisfy our hunger. Its workings remain geared to material comfort while our needs are elsewhere.

Bach's flower essences can help us put the focus where it belongs and meet those higher needs, so giving us that sense of continuous happiness and fulfilment. 'These remedies have assisted us to grow, to learn, to understand, to expand, to develop, to cope, to enjoy and to be, in a way that I never thought possible before,' says Liz Bailey, a practitioner on the Isle of Man. 'My sense of spirituality has completely opened up. The remedies are the food of the spirit when it hungers.'

downshifting

True abundant living has nothing to do with the size of our cars, houses and bank balances. It means fully experiencing every moment, learning as much as possible, being alert and centred in our lives. We can live abundantly with the bare necessities of existence by knowing when to move up the pyramid. Or we can stay stuck and live narrow lives surrounded by wealth. The truth of this is reflected in the phenomenon of downshifting.

Downshifting came to prominence in the 1990s as a reaction to the materialistic have-it-all 1980s. Some see it as an affluent phenomenon, a luxury that poor people can ill afford. Certainly it is easy and even fashionable to cut down from three to two foreign holidays or seek the simple life in expensive and beautifully appointed health clubs and retreats. But this is at best a half-truth. Gandhi wasn't rich, yet his teachings about the art of enjoying a life of renunciation make him the archetypal downshifter. And people who start with little are no more likely to resist the siren call of materialism. In Ecuador I knew a poor and hard-working family who claimed they could not afford to give their children fresh fruit and vegetables, yet still owned a twenty-four-inch colour television.

Downshifting means taking control of our lives by cutting back on the things and activities that possess us. We might buy fewer ready-prepared meals, not buy clothes unless we are going to wear them, not feel we need to change the car so often. We might leave a hated and remunerative job for one with less pay and more satisfaction. We might say 'no' to some opportunities in order to focus on the things that are really important to us. Downshifting could involve us in recycling our rubbish or going to the bottle bank or building a compost heap in the garden. We may grow some of our own food. We may cut our own hair or make our own wine. We may send back the video camera and spend our evenings keeping journals of our lives instead.

All these activities are worthwhile and can be part of a profound lifestyle change, but we shouldn't become so preoccupied with them that they become an end in themselves. Carried through with clear vision, downshifting is not a destination but a means to a more fulfilling life, a way of shifting up the pyramid and of moving towards self-development and self-transcendence. The exact pattern of life we will create for ourselves depends on who we are. Nevertheless, all downshifters will recognise the items on the following list as main areas of concern for which some kind of answer needs to be sought.

❁ **A closer relationship with nature.** Downshifters tend to spend more time in the natural world and less time in man-made environments. City-dwellers move to small towns and people in towns move into the countryside. Living off the land becomes an ideal. Spiritual satisfaction comes from growing food, collecting wood for fires, walking the earth. Activities that involve living things – plants, animals, whole environments – are valued more than activities involving manufactured objects.

❁ **A closer relationship with other human beings.** Downshifters consciously spend time with others. Family relationships and other personal bonds are prized and developed. Children are given space and time and encouragement. Beyond the immediate circle there is a sense of commitment to the community and to future generations.

❁ **Personal creativity.** Downshifters are committed to discovering and enhancing their creative potential. This can involve artistic activities such as painting, writing and music-making, but attention to creativity also expresses itself in everyday activities such as cooking and home-making.

❀ **Simplicity and quietness.** Successful downshifters are careful not to exchange the constant busyness of materialism for the constant busyness of thrift. They build space and time into their days so they have opportunities for thought and meditation. 'Simple living' must include 'just' living, time to be. If we are always engaged in doing then we are just re-creating the rat race in new surroundings.

❀ **Finding one's inner self.** Downshifters look for more meaningful activities than the ones they abandoned. This leads them to consider what special qualities and gifts they bring to life. They aim to cultivate their gifts and so discover and express their true selves rather than act out roles set up for them by society.

❀ **Balance and expression.** Downshifters are in touch with their feelings and able to express them honestly. They value their emotions and seek a point of balance where they can be in harmony with themselves and with the rest of the universe.

Goals like self-expression and finding one's true path in life have a clear relationship with Bach's system. In particular, the whole concept of emotional balance and empathy with others is central to what Edward Bach's flower essences do. 'People seem to slow down and take time to enjoy the simple pleasures in life when they are helped with the remedies,' says Linda Beckenham, an aromatherapist and reflexologist who uses Bach essences as a complement to her other therapies. 'I believe they learn to respect others once they have learned to respect themselves.'

i 🌺 courage

Fear is the main source of superstition, and one of the main sources of cruelty. To conquer fear is the beginning of wisdom.
– Bertrand Russell, English philosopher, in *Unpopular Essays*, 1950

groups

In 1936 Edward Bach presented his finished system in a booklet called *The Twelve Healers and Other Remedies*. In it he organised the thirty-eight essences under seven headings.

🌺 for *fear*
🌺 for *uncertainty*
🌺 for those *over-sensitive* to influences and ideas
🌺 for *insufficient interest* in present circumstances
🌺 for *loneliness*
🌺 for *despondency* or despair
🌺 for *over-care* for welfare of others

In chapters i to vii of *Bloom* we will examine the remedies in each of these groups and identify the positive potential of each. We will see how each flower helps resolve a particular emotional state and so has its own message for all of us engaged on a spiritual journey. The essences incarnate pure qualities – virtues, for want of a better word – that are

There is no other medicine that treats the emotional side of being human, which is what so many of us struggle with. They can be likened to a 'key of life', a tool to use at any time without fear of side effects or having to make an appointment. They are open to everyone who will see them. – Claire Bickerton

I no longer label some of the remedies 'awkward and just not for me'. All of them have been and will continue to be a wonderful tool to increase self-knowledge. – Catherine

central to our quest to become fully grown humans and live more abundantly. If we are suffering the negative aspects of a remedy that is both a sign that we need to develop the corresponding virtue, and an invitation to do so.

five remedies to give courage

Cowards die many times before their deaths;
The valiant never taste of death but once.
Of all the wonders that I yet have heard,
It seems to me most strange that men should fear;
Seeing that death, a necessary end,
Will come when it will come.
– William Shakespeare, *Julius Caesar*, Act 2, Scene 2

Shakespeare's Julius Caesar claimed not to understand fear, but he was something of a politician so we shouldn't take this at face value. For nature has wired fear into us. It is the most primitive of all emotions. While some scientists reject the idea that so-called 'lower' animals can feel social emotions like jealousy and disappointment, all recognise fear as a basic emotion common to all creatures from fish to hamsters to humans. Fear plays a crucial role in the flight-or-fight response that helps animals survive in the wild. It pumps blood to the leg muscles so that we can run away faster, and it freezes us for a moment first so that we have time to think about hiding instead. When a tiger was creeping up on one of our ancestors the ability to freeze, think of a safe place and run like hell was crucial to survival.

Fear remains helpful today when danger threatens, although most of the time its causes are more mundane. Moderate nerves just before speaking in public increase our adrenaline levels. We think and react faster and so turn in a better performance than the dead-calm dead-boring next person. The same goes for all those other well-known anxiety-inducers – sitting exams, taking tests, attending job interviews. A touch of apprehension can be a good thing; Julius Caesar might have sensed and avoided his imminent assassination if he had been a little less sure of himself.

To be useful, fear must be in proportion to the situation. We can represent the link between anxiety and performance using a bell curve. At the top of the curve, a moderate amount of anxiety gives the best possible performance; not enough anxiety and we perform poorly because we lack motivation to do our best; too much anxiety and we perform badly because we can't think straight. Instead of feeling alert and together we begin to look scared and ill at ease. Instead of thinking faster we begin to think of nothing but how afraid and uncomfortable we are. A similar bell curve applies to the time scale over which anxiety lasts. Feeling a little anxious just before a driving test is normal and helpful but the same level of anxiety in the six months leading up to the test isn't, nor is anxiety that continues after the test is over when we should be celebrating. Long-term anxiety is wearing on mind and body and causes a range of symptoms including a pale or flushed complexion, rapid pulse, decreased sexual drive, a tight chest, sweating, dizziness, light-headedness and that familiar sinking feeling in the pit of the stomach.

Balance doesn't mean never feeling anxious. Rather it means keeping anxiety in its place, so that it only comes when it is useful and doesn't take over our lives. When it is too frequent or too powerful fear stops us from taking risks and stops us from listening to our inner voice. We are as spontaneous as rabbits frozen in the fast lane headlights. We will only begin to move and act when we develop and express our qualities of courage, faith and resilience. This is what the essences in Bach's first group can help us do.

Bach identified five specific kinds of fear, and each has its corresponding flower.

❀ **Mimulus** gives quiet courage when we are afraid of specific things.
It also helps those of us who suffer from shyness and feel ill at ease
in company or when the spotlight is on us.

❀ **Rock Rose** unfreezes the rabbit. When great terror leaves us unable
to act or think coherently this is the flower to build our courage so
that we can face the worst trials with clear-sighted determination.

❀ **Aspen** gives us faith in the essential goodness and rightness of the
world. It helps us overcome vague fears that are not related to any
specific cause. Superstitious fears can also melt away with the help
of Aspen's grounded courage and confidence.

❀ **Cherry Plum** gives our conscious mind a greater sense of being
guided and under control, helping us to stay rational and focused
whatever the provocation.

❀ The people we love have their own lives to live and need to take risks
and trust themselves. **Red Chestnut** helps us calm any anxieties we
have about their welfare. We can radiate fearlessness and support
them through their mistakes by showing we believe in them.

Anxiety and fear are friends in some situations, enemies in others. But in
all cases they are invitations to rediscover the depths of our courage and
inner security. This is the right way to look at fear, so that it becomes an
opportunity rather than a problem. Fear, as Bach's assistant Nora Weeks
once pointed out, is simply a test of courage.

> I have not been accepting of the word 'fear'. I did not want to
> associate with such a negative concept. But I am re-evaluating my
> relationship to it. By being more honest with myself and bringing
> my fears up to the light, I see how much more quickly and pain-
> lessly I can understand what they are trying to teach me, learn
> from them, thank them, and let them dissolve. – Michael Hillier

face your fear: mimulus

Mimulus relates to the everyday fears of life, quiet fears, fears that we keep to ourselves or speak of to only a few people. Any fear for which we can name a cause is a Mimulus fear, and that includes everything from fear of poverty and illness and burglars and enclosed spaces right up to the fear of death itself, regardless of whether the fear is rational or not.

Mimulus is an especially important development aid for those of us who suffer from shyness. We may blush or stammer in company, or adopt a nervous laugh or a bluff manner to conceal our insecurity. We think of social events as a trial to be got through rather than a celebration to be enjoyed. 'I avoided using the telephone and often ignored it when it rang,' says Alice, who describes herself as a Mimulus type. 'If anyone so much as walked past the end of the drive my heart would grip with fear in case they were coming to the house. I lost contact with all my school friends and apart from my husband I remained friendless for about fifteen years. At work I was grateful I had little contact with others.' The flower helps us to overcome crippling anxieties of this kind without the need for pretence or embarrassment. It allows us to enjoy our lives and the company of others, which means in turn that we can be better friends to those around us and better integrated into our relationships and community.

We see positive Mimulus in the child standing up to bullies in the playground, or determinedly climbing the stairs in the dark, or dealing with her fear of high places, her phobia of spiders and her anxieties over making new friends. She is the quiet woman who unexpectedly speaks out against an injustice, or amazes her colleagues by giving a calm and witty speech at a conference. She is the reserved person whose understated humour gleams like gold at parties. Never seeking the limelight, she will not wilt when it turns towards her. In an emergency her poise and equanimity make her an invaluable and reliable friend.

I remember magpies swooping at me and pecking at my head when I was a child. All my life I was frightened of birds and terrified if one came near me. After a course of Mimulus my fear dissipated, and the courage I found enabled me to go into a fowl yard, collect eggs, touch birds and not panic when one came near me. – Rosemary Barry

I always wanted to mix with people, but was too shy to do so and so felt left out of things. It's only recently that I have accepted this part of my personality and looked at it from the positive side rather than the negative. Being a Mimulus has given me a sensitive side to my nature which is certainly a blessing. – J.C.

The smaller fears – of flying insects and climbing onto furniture to do the decorating – began to leave me. But the fear of being struck dumb with groups of people intensified for a while, as Mimulus brought the problem up into awareness. But Mimulus in hand, I have spoken in public on numerous occasions and have been employed as a lecturer. – Susan

I always worried about having an accident. Perhaps not so much the accident itself, but rather the thought of having to deal with the other driver and the police. I recognised myself as a Mimulus type. I had a short spell of feeling worse and fearing that perhaps I had to experience an accident in order to face it, so that I would learn that there was nothing to be afraid of. This passed and I began to enjoy driving. – Alice Walkingshaw

I started with Mimulus in November and noticed a very different feeling at my office Christmas party. I actually enjoyed it! There were some social occasions I always met with apprehension, this being one of them, but that year I was quite suddenly not 'me' – or, should I say, I *was ME*. – Jill Woods

I was an incredibly shy child who used to blush if anyone spoke to me or even looked at me. Even after teaching for twelve years it is still hard to stand up in front of a group of people, but I do it. I have learned how to manage my shyness. Mimulus played a great part in this development, which hasn't come overnight. It has helped me feel the fear and face it and stand my ground. – Helen Kent

courage to act: rock rose

The second remedy against fear is Rock Rose. It relates to the positive qualities of heroism and bravery. It helps us stay aware during emergencies and crises so we can find the strength and will to act, and choose our actions wisely and without fear of the consequences. Rock Rose risks her life if she needs to. She is the mother plunging into a river to save her drowning child: she has forgotten herself and is taking action to overcome the cause of a terror.

According to Bach, Rock Rose is the 'remedy of emergency for cases when there even appears no hope'. We take it when we feel paralysed with fear, unable to think coherently, or in such a panic that it is all we can do not to run away in terror. It is useful in times of great need and urgency, when we face death and destruction or are the victims of accidents. And we can also take it when we witness somebody else's terror. Panic spreads like fire and needs to be quenched wherever it appears. Even as bystanders our increased calmness and lack of fear can only help the person actually in the situation.

trust the good: aspen

According to legend the aspen tree has shaken with horror and remorse ever since the Romans used it to make the cross on which they crucified

Jesus. Only on Christmas Day does it stand still. Botanists have a more prosaic explanation for its constant rustle, and point to the long springy stalk that attaches its leaves to its branches, so that the slightest breath of air makes the leaves shiver. But the association with fear and horror is still there. In the Bach Centre garden, talking with somebody under the aspen tree, a breeze came and the tree whispered above and around us. 'I couldn't have this tree outside my house,' she said. 'I like quiet trees. This one is too creepy.'

Henry James Sr, father of the famous novelist, described going through an Aspen state in his 1879 book *Society, the Redeemed Form of Man*. Colin Wilson cites the passage in *The Outsider*, his exploration of existential unease, and the account is so graphic that it is worth repeating here.

> One day towards the close of May, having eaten a comfortable dinner, I remained sitting at the table after the family had dispersed [...] when suddenly – in a lightning flash, as it were – 'fear came upon me, and trembling made all my bones to shake.' To all appearances it was a perfectly insane and abject terror without ostensible cause, and only to be accounted for, to my perplexed imagination, by some damned shape, squatting invisible to me within the precincts of the room, and raying out from his fetid personality influences fatal to life.

James called this experience a 'vastation'. The word captures well the sense of helplessness that we feel when our fear comes from nowhere and in so doing seems out of the ordinary scale of things. If we are afraid of dogs or giving speeches we can avoid them or learn more about them. If we are afraid of nothing there seems nothing to be done.

In the Aspen state there is a vague dread, varying in intensity from a generalised foreboding – something creepy about the whispering leaves – to an extreme hair-on-end, shaking terror. In the Aspen state we feel that something is dreadfully wrong or that something terrible may happen at any moment, but we can't say what it is that we fear. Aspen fear is the terror felt on waking after a nightmare. The dream itself and the things we saw in it have been forgotten, but the fear remains.

The way beyond this experience, as Wilson points out, usually and perhaps necessarily requires some form of religious or philosophical accommodation with life. We need to believe in the essential goodness of the universe. We need to trust that whatever may happen it will help us grow and will never be more than we can cope with. This echoes the thinking of the Roman stoic Seneca. He had a peculiar way of comforting his friends when they were anxious. Instead of saying, 'There's nothing to worry about,' he would encourage them to imagine that the worst possible outcome was actually happening. 'There's nothing to worry about,' would only encourage them to think how awful it would be if something did happen. Thinking the thing through brought the realisation that the very worst, whatever it was, could be lived through. Things could be bad, but they would never turn out as bad as they seemed before they happened. Why give space and time to nameless fears? Name them, think through them, then let them go.

I wanted to leave the bookshop where I worked and start a new life adventure. But doubt kept holding me back. In the local health food shop I started chatting to the assistant about my dilemma and she suggested I take Mimulus for known fear and to gain courage, Larch to gain self-confidence and Aspen to conquer fear of the unknown. Within a month I began to feel more positive, gained the courage to follow my heart and leave the bookshop for a college course. I haven't looked back since. If I hadn't gone into the shop and met the woman who suggested the remedies, my path would have been totally different. – Helen Kent

Aspen is the flower of fearlessness and belief in goodness. She stands in a place of great stillness in which nothing can cause her to bow – not pain, or worry, or suffering – for she believes absolutely in the eventual triumph of love and faith. She is brave and adventurous because she fears no danger; she walks in the darkness and brings her own light with her. She has the gift of understanding. Secure in her inner self, she learns the nature of the things she fears and knows them as part of the whole and so part of herself. They can no longer stop her from moving forward.

stay sane: cherry plum

Expressing how we feel can help release lopsided emotions and get us back into balance. But it's a mistake to think that expressing emotions is the same as losing control. If we fall into the habit of always letting go, letting rip and letting it all hang out we become like habitual drunkards, possessed by what we have allowed into us and unable to rise above our feelings or understand their lesson. And if our feelings overwhelm us we can end up like children in a temper tantrum, unable to cope with what we have released and afraid of the strength of our own feelings. This is the negative Cherry Plum state – one in which the tiny 'I' is caught up and swept along in uncontrollable and irrational emotion. In this state we feel desperate, terrified, frantic for a way out. The mind is under great strain and threatens to give way. We are afraid we might do something crazy or out of character: hit our children, slap our partner, grab some weapon without stopping to think of the consequences. We may injure ourselves, or even take our own life. And again, the overriding feeling is one of fear: fear of losing our reason, our sanity, our very selves.

Sometimes the Cherry Plum state arrives out of the blue, resulting perhaps from a sudden crisis or acute physical pain. Bach actually discovered the remedy as a cure for a frantic state brought on by a sudden attack of sinusitis. Other times we crack under some long-standing pressure. Mild physical discomfort can leave us desperate if it goes on for long enough, as can any chronic social or mental or emotional pressure, such as poor housing conditions, poverty, a bad-tempered partner or pressure at work. Squabbling children are another everyday cause. All parents will recognise the moment when we are so desperate for quiet and rationality that we have to hold ourselves in to prevent ourselves from hurting our children.

Even if we are successful at repressing the storms and not showing the cracks we still have the fear of cracking, and this too is a negative. Better by far to find a way of building up our reserves of sanity and self-possession so that we will not snap and don't need to fear doing so. Cherry Plum opens to us this better path. It resolves the negative state by bringing the small and terrified 'I' back into contact with that well-spring of calm and security that Bach called the higher self. This allows us to express our emotions in a positive way. For the cleanest release of emotion comes when we remain rational and coherent. Only then can we consciously let go of our negative feelings, put them in context, learn from them and choose to move forward.

> Six of us were living in two small caravans while waiting to build our house. We were fighting planning appeals against a consortium of neighbours. I was drinking far too much and felt I was losing control and heading for a nervous breakdown. I didn't know what I might do next – perhaps do or say something to the neighbours that I would regret, also to my partner who I thought had deserted me. Cherry Plum was my first remedy, among others. After a couple of weeks I was able to acknowledge these desperate feelings and find a balance. I moved out of this irrational state that had blocked me so totally. – Claire Hingley

radiate courage: red chestnut

In the *Illustrated Handbook of the Bach Flower Remedies* Philip Chancellor tells how Bach discovered the Red Chestnut remedy:

> Dr Bach had a bad accident with an axe; this caused great anxiety on the part of those close to him as immediate first aid was applied to stanch the blood. When he had recovered, Dr Bach said that [they] had experienced the state of mind of the next remedy which he would seek; a remedy to counteract the fear for others. He also added that [their] anxiety on his behalf, although [they] had done [their] best to hide it, had not helped him at all. His sensitivity was so great that he could not avoid sensing and reacting to [their] feelings of the moment.

All of us sense and react to other people's feelings to some extent, and of all the emotions anxiety is the most catching. We are programmed at a primitive level to be on the look-out for danger. If our friend looks scared then we get scared too; and if our friend is nervous about our ability to cope with something we too become anxious and lose our confidence and self-belief. Imagine a teenager going to a late-night party for the first time. If her father is anxious and insists that she call home every hour she will not be able to enjoy the experience for what it is. Her thoughts and feelings will be skewed towards his. She will end up anxious herself.

If we are being worried over and need protection from this the essence to use is Walnut; we will meet this flower in chapter iii. If we are the worrier we need the fear remedy Red Chestnut. This helps us keep calm about other people's problems and experiences. It reminds us that all of us are working out different patterns in life and that somebody putting herself at risk may be walking a necessary part of her path. Our world would be poorer if concerned friends of Florence Nightingale had managed to infect her with their anxiety. Red Chestnut gives us confidence that the people we love will be able to rise to the challenges they face, like she did. And just as we can touch others with our anxiety and make them in turn anxious, so we will spread our new feelings of security and confidence to those we love. With the help of Red Chestnut the teenager's dad will be a centre of stability and reassurance for his child. If she does get into trouble and call home for advice he will be able to act calmly so as to give her what she needs. And what she needs is never somebody else's fear.

> After my mother's too early death I became obsessively worried about other family members, and sometimes felt acute anxiety. Red Chestnut gradually helped me to calm down.
> – Nobuko Asanuma

change and fear

Try this exercise if you feel comfortable with it. Pick a time when you won't be interrupted by friends or family or pets, and take the phone off the hook before you begin.

1. Lie down in a dark and quiet room.
2. Close your eyes and listen to your breathing. Allow your breath to slow gradually and feel yourself relax.
3. When you are comfortable and calm think about your body. Imagine it as something made up of elements, of countless atoms. Think about those atoms and their relationship to the rest of the universe. Imagine the journey your atoms will take in the future, into elements, into plants and then into animals and new human beings.

4. You are completely relaxed now. Imagine the atoms of your body returning to the earth. You are falling away from your life and dying. It is a completely peaceful and natural thing to do and you feel unafraid and happy.

5. Think about your life energy and its journey into whatever you believe, whether up to heaven or back into the eternal field of force that nets the universe. Feel this journey as good and natural and part of the dance of life.

6. Go back to your breathing and listen to it continue as you come back into life. When you are ready, open your eyes.

This should be a peaceful and rewarding moment. If you feel any fear or discomfort at any point, come out of it and take the fear remedy or remedies you need.

One advantage of this exercise is that it helps us accept our eventual and inevitable death as a positive moment of change. It gives us a little of Caesar's equanimity without requiring the same degree of ignorance; Seneca would have approved. Another is that accepting the idea and necessity of death makes it easier to accept the necessity of the little deaths that occur throughout life – losing old habits, old friends, old environments. We change all the time, and every change is an opening out of new possibilities. Viewing changes in this way, not with a blind and total lack of fear but with a fully conscious confidence in our ability to overcome fear, puts us in a good position from which to evolve.

2 ❀ evolution

emotions and rationality

In general emotions arise from the older parts of the brain, the limbic system and brainstem, which go right back to the early evolution of mammalian life. Pure intellect has more to do with the neocortex, which only appeared a hundred million years ago. The neocortex allows us to think about and rationalise and if necessary override our emotional responses. It also allows us to have *meta-emotions* – feelings about the way we feel – and so adds subtlety to our emotional life. Left to itself the old brain would be prey to strong passions. The new brain makes control and reflection possible, as well as a deeper and more profound emotional life that can experience altruism and empathy beyond the needs of evolutionary survival.

For most of the last 200 years orthodox medicine and society as a whole were firmly on the side of the neocortex, and tended to under-value feeling in the name of reason. Society taught its children to repress their passions, and considered open displays of affection or dislike impolite and a sign of poor breeding. When our emotions boiled over into inappropriate behaviour doctors suppressed them with drugs or used the more reductive forms of psychoanalysis to drain them of power. Even today calling somebody 'cool', meaning cold, impassive and impervious to feeling, is a way of giving praise.

These old-fashioned and fashionable attitudes are disappearing as we come to realise that emotions and reason are not opposites but complements. The emerging picture is of a balanced brain in which our feelings about things actually form the basis of rational choice. As Daniel Goleman shows in his book *Emotional Intelligence*, the theory that the brain is a computer falls to bits when we understand that a computer, with no sense of personal preference and no system of emotional values, would find it impossible to make a sensible decision over which tie to wear, which sentence to write next, which football team to support, or who to marry. If our limbic system didn't have its preferences, its likes and dislikes, we wouldn't be able to make these decisions either. Without feelings about life reason would be adrift on a limitless tide of pros and cons, with a counter-argument washing against every argument and no paddle with which to steer. Emotions and values are inextricably linked. Reason alone could justify fascism and the police state as a rational solution to the problem of government. But almost all of us look at oppressive government and *feel* it is wrong. Our emotions – our gut feelings – tell us that liberty and freedom from state control override the need for ordered streets and the timely arrival of trains.

Goleman quotes many studies that show how overall intelligence and ability increase when we are fully aware of our feelings. But awareness alone is not enough if it begins and ends with the admission made by Andrea, a university lecturer: 'Sometimes I'm irritable or moody with people I care about,' she says. 'I know I'm being horrible but I don't seem able to stop it.' We can't learn from our lives if we are in the grip of unbalanced negative feelings, any more than we can learn from emotional blindness. Both states hinder our ability to see patterns and deal better with our environments and opportunities.

For Andrea and for all of us the next step after awareness is control: being able to stop it. But the kind of control we need is not the repression of drugs and the stiff upper lip. Instead it is a more flexible art, close cousin to the skills of a talented rider who uses empathy and understanding to channel her horse in positive ways, and values him as a friend and partner rather than treating him as a beast to be broken, tied down or shut in a cage. Balance means having appropriate emotions: not so dim that we barely feel at all, not so out of control that they take away our ability to learn and grow. Instead of damping down feelings the holistic approach would be to bring emotions and rationality back into this kind of harmonious relationship. Both are necessary if we are to move without unnecessary struggle towards personal and spiritual growth. 'I was brought up not to express emotions or feelings, so discovering the Bach flower remedies has been a most beautiful and revealing experience for me,' says Beth, a practitioner who works with both horses and people. Another, Susanne, feels the same. 'Since I started using the remedies I am much more aware of my feelings and different moods,' she says. The result has been dramatic. 'I feel my life has changed one hundred per cent. I believe I have found my true self and my centre of harmony within me.' Like so many Bach practitioners, Beth and Susanne now help others with something that helped them in the past.

balance and evolution

According to evolutionary biologists common physical symptoms such as fever and morning sickness bring clear benefits to the human beings who suffer them. Fevers raise the body temperature to a degree that is uncomfortable for invading bacteria and viruses, so helping the body to resist them. Morning sickness tends to make highly spiced, strong and bitter foods like coffee, alcohol and some herbs less appealing, and these are precisely the foods that can harm the developing foetus. Taking drugs to control fevers and morning sickness can therefore be counter-productive. The lowered body temperature allows the viruses to multiply; the absence of nausea allows the consumption of dangerous foods.

If unpleasant physical symptoms can be good and desirable, what about unpleasant emotional symptoms? Beyond the role normal emotions play in rational thought, could there be an on-going evolutionary benefit to be had from anxiety or depression or apathy?

Clearly it's easier to think of an evolutionary advantage for some emotions than it is for others. Anxiety is simple, up to a point. If we run a mile at every noise we will not get eaten by a tiger and will live to breed another day. Fear of snakes and spiders makes us less likely to get bitten by a poisonous animal. But apathy is harder to justify – apathetic people are less alert and will be made a meal of more often. Using the Darwinian model we might expect apathy to have been bred out of humanity a long time ago. What evolutionary advantage might we gain from feeling depressed or despondent when things go wrong, especially given the negative effects these states have on our physical health and ability to reproduce? I am not convinced by theorists who suggest that depression might be a deterrent aimed at stopping us from repeating an unsuccessful piece of behaviour, especially as trying again at once is so often a successful strategy, as we discover when we are teenagers looking for a dance partner at parties. It's even harder to find a justification for genuinely out-of-control emotions like chronic anxiety and endogenous depression. The kind of fear that leads us to run from shadows and moving leaves will get in the way of eating, sleeping and other important activities including breeding. If depression is not caused by an external factor like a setback, where is the advantage in our continued brooding? Orthodox medicine agrees, and seeing no advantage in these states seeks to suppress them using tranquillisers and antidepressants in the same way it uses drugs to suppress fever.

Edward Bach would not agree with this. In his model of life all kinds of negative emotions have a part to play in evolution, although the evolution he was talking about was not Darwinian. The latter is the result of blind natural forces, a succession of small changes from generation to generation based on an individual's ability to reproduce and create offspring. Bach talked about evolution as a spiritual process that took place through the single lifetime of an individual. Furthermore he saw evolution as teleological: in other words, it had an end in view. In Darwinian evolution we evolve away from things that threaten and kill us. Bach believed we evolve towards something: the perfection of the individual self.

fundamental considerations

Bach spelt out his ideas about personal spiritual evolution in an essay called 'Some Fundamental Considerations of Disease and Cure', which he published in the journal *Homoeopathic World* in 1930. He starts by separating the individual into two parts. On the one hand is the manifestation of a human being on earth. This includes physical matter – blood, bone and flesh – but also the human mind, ego and personality. This worldly part is the first and least important part of a human being. Of greater importance is the spiritual self or soul, the second part, which Dr Bach often referred to as the higher self. The higher self incarnates itself on earth through the personality and the body, but is not dependent on them and pre-exists and survives the life of the body. The higher self wants to express perfection in the physical world. The role of the personality on earth is to help the higher self achieve this. It learns and develops during its physical life, with the aim of reaching perfection in the flesh.

We tend to think of happiness as a goal, a static thing or place at the end of a road. In the common view of heaven, for example, the journey is a struggle, but having got there we stop struggling and lie around being happy for all eternity. This is the idea of happiness that George Bernard Shaw had in mind when he made one of his characters say, 'I don't want to be happy; I want to be alive and active.' But as we saw when we looked at Abraham Maslow's hierarchy of needs, real happiness is a process, not a state, and being alive and active and growing up the pyramid are part of being happy. In Bach's model happiness comes when the personality is developing and growing under the soul's direction. As long as the personality is fulfilling the higher self's aims then all is joy, says Bach. Happiness accompanies every stage of our development, regardless of what stage we have reached. We may not all reach enlightenment but if we choose to move towards it and be active and alive we will certainly be happy. The way of growth open to us is 'a slow, gradual and should be happy evolution'. But by the same token if we lose touch with the spiritual self we are diminished, no matter how high up the pyramid we have climbed. In Bach's memorable phrase we become 'an empty shell, a cork upon the waters'. This leaves us susceptible to attack by the ever-present physical agents of disease such as viruses, physical breakdown and bacteria. Indeed, Bach believed that disease could sometimes be a 'corrective' sent by the higher self to discourage us from going down the wrong path.

We again hear the early rumbles of Maslow's later theories when Bach describes how each individual human life traces a similar course of evolution. As babies we start with basic physical needs for warmth, food and shelter. As the personality develops we move towards worldly desires for money, power, possessions and sex. But the real work of our life on earth begins when we start to think about the needs of others and to see our lives in relationship to other lives and to life itself. This is when things get tough, because spiritual success on earth means that we have to turn our selfish and worldly desires inside out. We have to turn away from greed and materialism and towards a kind of divine selflessness.

As well as working on our overall spiritual evolution Bach found that we tend to have one particular virtue that we need to develop through the course of our lifetime. Different people will be working on different virtues. The situation in which we find ourselves guides us to what 'our' virtue is: as Bach says, 'we are not placed in the luxury of a palace to overcome hardship bravely: nor do we come as paupers to learn the wise control of wealth.' (Incidentally, Bach tacitly accepts the concept of reincarnation in this essay. Another more explicit reference is in his later book *Heal Thyself* where he talks of our 'previous and later life, apart from this present one'. He believed that a single soul will incarnate many times in order to express the many virtues it has to develop.)

George Harrison, always the most spiritually inclined of the Beatles, once said in an interview that we 'don't become God-conscious in half an hour'. Bach says the same thing. The greatest changes come over time, and we can't force the pace of development. So we don't have to renounce everything and live in a nunnery to find our spiritual path, or experience some blinding and dramatic revelation, and the chances are that neither is the right path for us anyway. Most of us can learn more from raising children and earning a living than from sitting in a cell contemplating. Wherever we are now that is where our path can be found. We can change slowly and learn at our own pace, little by little.

Change and growth are rarely constant. Sometimes we move forward, sometimes we stand still – and if we feel unhappy that is a sure sign that we have got stuck. Early in his research Bach wondered if the cause of an emotional blockage might be indicated by the kind of physical symptom a person suffered from: if people with heart problems, for example, might have problems loving others. He abandoned this theory when he realised that heart trouble, like any other physical problem, can as easily result from overwork or anxiety. In his later writings he was clear that the emotions themselves are the clearest guide to the underlying problem. Feelings of impatience or aggression or fright are direct indicators of the positive potentialities that are not being sufficiently developed. If we get bogged down in our worries and can no longer hear the problems of others that means we need to work on our ability to empathise with other people. This *is* the task that we have been set by our higher self. If we choose essences to overcome that negative emotion they help us to develop the virtue that is lacking, making it easier for us to get back on course and achieve the next step.

Bach believed that overcoming and transmuting negative emotions and the other obstacles life puts in our path was the very aim of evolution. In his view, then, it is only partially correct to say that we evolved into anxious people so as to avoid tigers. It is just as true to say that the negative is there to give us something to strive against, that anxiety helps us to develop courage. Negatives turn out to be positive. They help us develop virtue in the same way weights build up strength. By moving beyond anger, hatred, indolence and despair we find new and immortal qualities in ourselves. We turn from self to self-lessness, from separation to unity, from negative to positive. Bad feelings and difficulties are our servants because they help us identify areas for development. We need to welcome them, explore them, read their message, and with the help of the flower essences, do something about them. 'Issues I found difficult started to appear normal when I began using the remedies,' says Aneeta, who works out of a health clinic in Bombay and started using the essences in the late 1980s. 'I no longer panicked or felt resentful when faced with problems. I learned to accept life and its processes. I gained clarity of thought and stability, and discovered inner strength to find equilibrium in my life.'

utopias, spin and gravity

From Plato to Thomas More to nineteenth-century socialists like William Morris and Edward Bellamy, writers have felt obliged to people their fictional utopias with ciphers. Perhaps this is because real people would never have agreed to live in any of them. While all of us would say that we want to be happy and in balance this doesn't mean that we all fit into the same ready-made boxes. Down here in the messy, muddy world balance means as many different things as there are different people. It is one thing to Ghandi, another to J.S. Bach, and something else again to you and to me. Yet we can still identify two qualities shared by all balanced people, and they are qualities that in themselves explain why utopias always fail, because both determine difference.

❀ **The first quality is to have found and worked at the thing in life that we love**. Our mission in life could be nursing or gardening or stock car racing or motherhood or fatherhood or a series of smaller commitments. Some of us are here to run businesses, some to run races, and the only right track is the one that brings us happiness.

❧ **The second quality is always to be ourselves**. Our natural personality – described in remedy terms as our *type remedy* – reflects how our evolutionary goals or the needs of our higher self differ. The different personality types have different centres of gravity so that when we balance we do so in different ways and spin at different rates. A balanced Centaury person will never be the same as a balanced Vervain.

These two factors are major influences on what that abstract idea 'a balanced life' will actually look and feel and taste and smell and sound like when we personally achieve it. We can't know where our path leads in advance and so we shouldn't allow our preconceptions to get in the way. We may turn out to be different from the way we assumed we were (we discover a hidden heart to our character) or to have a different role in life (an unexpected talent or opportunity opening a door).

The situation is even more complex and fluid than this sketch suggests. We are more than a simple, straightforward personality. Our idea of being in balance changes over time just as our needs and circumstances and moods change. Things happen and knock us off course. Achieving balance is not, therefore, a one-off effort that leaves us beyond history and unchanging for ever, and balance is not a finished artefact, something we do and then move on from. Instead, living a balanced life is an on-going commitment, a lifelong series of small choices that we make anew every day. It is natural and alive and growing, a process and a journey rather than a product and a goal. This leads to a position where we come back to flower essences – or any other balancing techniques we learn – at various points in our lives, as new issues come up and we work to overcome them. One person who does just this is Karen, a human resources consultant in the south-east of England. 'Taking the remedies helps by bringing up the concerns and issues I need to consider,' she says. 'I have moved from Elm to Vine to Beech to Impatiens to Agrimony to Rock Water.

Impatiens with Beechy moments is where I am at present, with dashes of Crab Apple coming up.'

Another remedy user's experience illustrates a point I made in an earlier book when I described the action of the remedies as *restorative* rather than *aspirational*. Susan started using Bach essences fifteen years ago on the advice of a friend. 'At the beginning I hoped the remedies would provide me with the positive traits I desired, as if plucked out of the air,' she says. 'But over the last few years I have come to understand that the remedies are drawing forth what is within me. People speak of me as having inner calm and a calming influence upon them. I believe this is due to the remedies drawing forth what is uniquely me.' As Susan's example shows, taking a flower does not change us into somebody different. Nor does it carry out spiritual development on our behalf, while we sit by and let it happen. What it does is put us back on track, back towards that central point of balance where we are more in line with our higher self and can once more take up our main task of learning from our life and carrying out our mission. The essences *restore* us to ourselves. 'I know I'm being horrible but I don't seem able to stop it,' said Andrea: the remedies are one way to stop being horrible and get back to being who we really are.

Once we get back to ourselves we are never in exactly the same place. Like a gyroscope knocked across a table top, we recover our balance and spin again in our own way, but we have moved. Suffering the negative emotion and overcoming it guarantees that we make progress – in Bach's terms, guarantees that we evolve. Having experienced the evil of depression, fear or loss of will we don't simply go back to a state of happy ignorance. Like Adam, we live our Fall. So despite being *restorative* there is nothing *conservative* about the essences. They don't take us back to the past, to who we used to be. They take us back to the present, to who we are, now that we have had this experience. They help us learn more effectively and move on. They help us take the next step to becoming who we can be. The remedies restore, and it is we ourselves who aspire.

ii ✿ decision and indecision

Sow an act, and you reap a habit. Sow a habit, and you reap a character.
Sow a character, and you reap a destiny.

– saying attributed to Charles Reade, nineteenth-century writer and
  dramatist

> Getting to know the philosophy behind the remedies made me
> look at them in a new light. They became more than just another
> alternative product. They are the only substance I know that
> gently touches the core of our being, making real and lasting
> difference to our lives. – Catherine

six remedies to sow an act

Life is learning, taking opportunities, taking action. But before we can act
we need to make plans, and to make plans we need to have a sense of
certainty: belief in our ability to look and move forward, confidence that
we are choosing the right action at the right time. Every plan we make
and every action we take presupposes that sense of certainty. Without it
we feel lost, confused, exhausted, despondent, and give up before starting or at the first setback. These are the times when Edward Bach's six
essences against uncertainty can help us.

- ✿ **Wild Oat** gives us certainty about our life's path. It helps when we
  struggle to discover what it is that we are born to do in life.
- ✿ **Scleranthus** relates to decisions big and small. It helps us hear our
  intuition and know our own minds and so put an end to dithering.

✿ **Cerato** comes into play when we know what is right for us but still ask for opinions and advice and so get led astray. Cerato helps us to be sure about our decisions.

✿ **Hornbeam** strengthens willpower at those moments when a task seems too much effort. It helps us get started and reminds us of the immense power that is ours to use.

✿ **Gentian** and **Gorse** are remedies for different stages of despondency. Gentian helps when we doubt our ability to overcome a setback. Gorse is for a deeper state in which we have chosen pessimism and feel that nothing can be done to help us.

purpose and freedom

Writing of her experiences in East Africa and her work with chimpanzees, the environmentalist and naturalist Jane Goodall breathes fulfilment. 'This is where I belong,' she says. 'This is what I came into this world to do.'

We are blessed when we know what our lives are for. One might play the piano, another sing or give herself up to organic gardening or ecological activism, another spend her time nursing others or raising children or creating a business or playing tennis or the stock market. There can be more depth and value in a life spent selling shoelaces – if that is what feels right – than in building houses or founding a church if those things feel wrong. The feeling – wrong or right – is more important than the activity. Our life has to fit us; if it doesn't it is never really ours. Other people's value judgements – 'you mean you want to sell *shoelaces*?' – are obstacles and not guides to the best way forward. If we walk it with conviction every path can lead to fulfilment.

The reason the feeling of rightness is so crucial is that it gives us a reason to act. Meaningful choice flows from value. If playing the piano feels right it needs no further analysis. It has intrinsic value, and at once becomes the source of all kinds of positive actions and decisions. If we find no intrinsic value in anything (if nothing feels right) there is no point in making choices and the concept of freedom loses meaning. In Bach's scheme identifying what feels right means contacting our higher self. The higher self knows what our mission is while the earth-bound personality may not have any clear idea of it; perhaps because it is not developed enough to understand the purpose, or perhaps because understanding the purpose is in fact the personality's whole task. Working in accordance with the higher self, our personalities gain freedom because they have a reason to act. Freedom is obeying the higher self.

> My growing acquaintance with the remedies has been a journey of self-discovery and self-knowledge. My awareness of my inner self and my soul's purpose has increased. Through the remedies I have begun my journey to true healing. – Martine Eyre

decide what: wild oat

In agriculture *sowing wild oats* meant making a mistake and sowing low-yield wild grains instead of high-yield cultivated grains. By extension the phrase came to mean spending youthful energy on riotous living and pleasure instead of getting on with the serious business of life. Some of the idea of making a mistake remains – we would have reaped more profit if we had been sober from the start – but there is no moral censure involved. Everybody starts out with some wild oats in hand. Better to sow them when we are young and have the time and energy to get over our excesses. Afterwards, calmer and more experienced, we should be in a better frame of mind to plot our course into adulthood. Perhaps Bach had these metaphorical wild oats in mind when he named his remedy for lack of direction in life, for the name is more poetic than factual. The Wild Oat remedy is not made from an oat at all, wild or otherwise, but from a type of grass whose Latin name is *Bromus ramosus*.

In a negative Wild Oat state we know we want to do *something* worthwhile in life but can't make up our minds what that *something* should be. So we try one thing after another and become more and more frustrated as we fail to find the sense of fulfilment that we are looking for. The typical Wild Oat person tries a number of different jobs, religions, lifestyles or philosophies but feels uncommitted to any of them and abandons them when they don't feel right. As she gets older she may get increasingly disillusioned and unhappy, and feel despair at the idea that she has missed her chance of living a worthwhile life.

The remedy helps us get a clearer idea of where our true path lies. It provides a signpost when we are lost and unsure where to go and points us back to our point of intrinsic value. Clearly Wild Oat is a central remedy in Bach's whole system, for more than any other it can be a key to finding happiness and fulfilment and a sense of purpose and growth. 'Your work is to discover your work, and then with all your heart to give yourself to it,' said Buddha. The literature of flower essences is full of tales of people who have used this remedy and in so doing have found their work and the right path to follow.

Up to the point I took Wild Oat the ideas I had concerning the rest of my life had been a mishmash of different thoughts with no coherence or path. The first change I noticed was that they were slowly coalescing into a cogent and formed plan.
– Jeff Chambers

I had been a nurse for eighteen years, and had an increasing urge to change direction in life without being entirely sure which way to turn. A teacher talked about Wild Oat during a workshop, so I started taking it as soon as I got home. Within six weeks I started training as an aromatherapist. I was given one of the last places on a course that had been delayed for two months. – Elaine

My husband and I were unhappy living in Edinburgh after ten years and were thinking about downshifting and moving to the country. We started taking Wild Oat to help us find our way and in a few months we offered on a property in the country. Now we have left the city and are happy living at the foot of a small glen in Perthshire. – Deirdre Barron

what decides?

At the University of California a researcher called Benjamin Libet sat some people in a room and attached electrodes to them. Then he asked them to bend one of their fingers whenever they wanted to. While they were doing this he measured three different points in time.

❀ *First*, the moment when the person consciously decided to bend a finger.

❀ *Second*, the moment the brain's electrical activity showed that a finger was about to bend.

❀ *Third*, the moment at which the finger actually moved.

He found that people's fingers moved one-fifth of a second after they had consciously decided to move them. But he also found that the brain started the moving process even earlier – a full third of a second *before* the person had actually decided to bend the finger. In other words, the unconscious mind was making the decision by itself, before the conscious mind became aware of it. The person's conscious 'decision' to move the finger at a particular time was not in fact the cause of the action. It was only a noticing of and agreement with a decision that had already been taken.

Libet's findings blow a giant hole in common assumptions about decision-making. They prove what psychologists have long suspected, that our judgements are not conscious and rational but instead come from far back in our minds. The job of the conscious mind is to find reasons to support decisions, or reconsider and abort them before they can be carried out. Our minds work like a parliament divided into two chambers: the first making policy and law; the second rubber-stamping it or sending it back for revision or throwing it out altogether. This is healthy and right, both in government and in our heads. In an ideal state first thoughts would need no revision – would in fact be the perfectly intuitive approach that Bach aspired to – but in our earth-bound reality decision-making is rarely perfect first time round, any more than we are ourselves. Unconscious decisions can result from prejudice and the machinations of the ego rather than the clean leading of intuition. We need the conscious moment of revision in order to avoid mistakes and damage to ourselves and to those around us.

Like any process, the conscious revision of first thoughts can get out of hand, so that we end up doubting and revising all our insights and ideas and throw out the baby of intuitive good feeling along with the bath-water of bigotry and self-interest. When this happens we fall into one of two lamentable states. Either we vacillate between our options, unable to settle among the endless pros and cons, or we lose all faith in our ability to do the right thing and start to ask other people for *their* opinions. In remedy terms, we either fall into Scleranthus or into Cerato.

decide how: scleranthus

Fourteen years ago I decided to go to a New Year's Eve party being given by the parents of a friend instead of going to the pub or to see a band. As a result of going to that party I got married, moved to the country, had three children and started working with Bach flower essences. If I hadn't gone to that party I would not be writing this book.

With hindsight we can all trace our current lives back to pivotal moments in the past, although at the time we had no way of knowing those moments would turn out to be pivotal. For me fourteen years ago deciding to go to the party was just one among a thousand either-ors that I weighed that day; so no doubt were the pivotal points in your own life. The important thing was that we made each trivial decision when the time came and didn't get too caught up in the process. For if we make choices smoothly and in a flowing way we are more likely to choose paths that feel intuitively right. And the paths that feel right are more likely to lead to higher and more meaningful goals. This is what Scleranthus helps us to do. If Wild Oat helps us decide what we want to aim at in life, Scleranthus helps us to get there turn by turn, intuitively, and without unnecessary angst.

In a negative Scleranthus state unconscious decisions get trapped in the conscious mind and ping backwards and forwards, from one option to another. First this way seems right, then the other, then we are back to the first. Often our indecision is over small things. We might be going to the theatre and spend an hour laying out sets of clothes – should we wear green or blue? – boots or shoes? – a belt or braces? – this or that pair of trousers? If we are enjoying this process and savouring it as good in itself, fine, there is no need for a remedy. But if we are tortured by the inability to decide Scleranthus can help us get a grip on the situation and make a choice, ideally before the curtain goes up.

The green or blue, boots or shoes examples suggest that Scleranthus is basically about choosing between two options. This is often true but is by no means a rule. There can be more than two alternatives. If we can't choose between green, blue and red that too is a Scleranthus decision, as is not being able to decide which of 400 T-shirts to buy. And Scleranthus can come into play when we consider weightier topics. Not knowing whether to marry Tom or Roger can be a Scleranthus problem if the goal – a good marriage – feels right but we aren't sure how best to get to it. On the other hand not being sure that marriage or anything else will bring us fulfilment is to do with our path in life and so would be a Wild Oat problem. With the more important life decisions, choosing between these two remedies can depend on how we frame the problem: is it about feeling ultimately unsatisfied with all the options (Wild Oat) or about choosing between directions that both seem right for different reasons (Scleranthus)?

People in a Scleranthus state don't usually ask for advice, but they sometimes express their fundamental indecision in other ways. Mood swings, erratic behaviour and lack of concentration might all be rooted in Scleranthus indecisiveness. In all such cases Scleranthus helps us hear again the small voice of right feeling so we can get back into balance and choose calmly and with certainty among the many ways open to us.

> Periodically I suffer from motion sickness and have found that Scleranthus does wonders for this. It has made me think about the reason for the nausea: might it have been a journey that part of me did not want to undertake, or a visit to someone I did not really want to spend time with? – Christine Philp

> I was planning a holiday visit to my eldest son who was living abroad. I couldn't decide whether to fly out or travel overland by rail. I agonised constantly over this decision, weighing up the pros and cons, until I decided to try Scleranthus. After three days of taking it regularly I suddenly realised that the whole idea was wrong, and that for various reasons I really shouldn't be going on this trip at all. I felt as though a great weight had been lifted from me, and I was able to get on happily with other plans and activities. – Helen

trust your judgement: cerato

The acorn, carried hundreds of miles from its mother tree, knows without instruction how to become a perfect oak. The fish of the sea and rivers lay their spawn and swim away. The same with the frog.

The serpent lays its eggs in the sand, and goes on its journey; and yet within the acorn, and the spawn, and the eggs is all the knowledge necessary for the young to become as perfect as their parents.

Young swallows can find their way to their Winter quarters hundreds of miles away, whilst parent birds are still busy with the second brood.

We need so much to come back to the knowledge that within ourselves lies all truth. To remember that we need seek no advice, no teaching but from within.

Edward Bach

When Bach started looking for healing flowers he excluded cultivated plants from consideration. Instead he looked for native or naturalised plants that grew wild in the countryside. In rising above their sometimes impoverished environments wild plants would prove their innate vigour and life force and so be a stronger basis for a healing remedy than something forced to grow using artificial means. He believed too that nature would provide true healing just as she provided all humanity's needs. There should be no need for human beings to 'create' healers by controlled propagation or cultivation.

Why then did Bach choose *Ceratostigma willmottiana* as raw material for a remedy? It's an unlikely choice, because cerato doesn't grow wild in England and Wales. Yet when he came across it in a garden in a Norfolk seaside village he asked the owner of the house for permission to take some of the flowers and from them prepared a remedy. After the event some doubt seemed to remain in his mind. Its rarity would make it difficult for his readers to find and prepare, a real worry at a time when only a handful of London pharmacies stocked remedies and people had to make their own. 'Cerato is not a native of this country and is only to be found on one or two private estates,' he wrote. 'It may later be possible to find a British substitute for this.' In fact he never did find a British substitute. Instead the plant he used grew in popularity. It is now quite easy to find.

Bach's discovery of the Cerato remedy is a good illustration of its power. In a negative Cerato state we know what we want because our intuition is leading us in the right direction (Bach prepared the flowers he found in somebody's garden despite their not matching what he was consciously looking for). But as soon as we have made our decision the doubts set in (having prepared the remedy he expressed doubt as to its suitability). The only thing missing from the story is the Cerato person's need to ask other people for their advice. In a classic Cerato state we ask a lot of questions. We actively seek out alternatives to our decision. We approach family, friends, work colleagues – even strangers at parties – and ask them what *they* would do if they were us. We receive all kinds of different advice, because other people are not us and have their own paths in life and their own intuitions and self-interest upon which to base their judgements. The longer this condition goes on the harder it is for us to hear our intuition telling us what to do, and the more likely it is that we will end up doing something quite different from what we wanted and quite different from what we need.

When Nora Weeks was at the Bach Centre she often had people come to her in a Cerato state, asking for guidance and direction. Her response was always the same: 'I can help you select the remedies you need, and they can help you in your current uncertainty, but I can't live your life for you. You must take your own decisions.' This is the message of Cerato. The flower gives us faith in our decisions and helps us trust that inside we know what is best for us. We have no need to ask other people for their opinions, for the opinion that really matters is the quiet voice within that guides us. In the end Bach kept to his decision. Cerato was never replaced and when he completed his researches in 1935 no doubt remained. This was the right flower and its place in the system was secure.

choose to start: hornbeam

We have all had moments when we feel that it will be physically and mentally impossible to take the next step. We have laid out the morning's work and then, at the moment to begin, feel weariness steal over us. It seems impossible to find the impetus to get going. Our strength fades along with our will. And yet as soon as we find the initial spark of energy the task assumes its usual proportions and we finish it before we realise. 'None of us is given more than we can accomplish,' wrote Bach, 'nor are we asked to do more than is within our power.' If this is true of our spiritual journey through life then it must also hold good for our everyday tasks.

Sometimes we are quick to find the needed spark within us. We spit on our hands, square our shoulders, and begin. All it takes is the first effort, the decision to start. Other times we look for something to distract us. The writer sitting down ready to write decides to check his e-mail first. (This is me, doing this.) Instead of ironing that shirt or digging the garden we make a cup of coffee or read the TV guide. We might give it up for the day and make some excuse. 'I'll do this tomorrow,' we say and 'this', whether it is filling in a form, learning a language or starting to meditate, is put off day by day as tomorrow turns into next week or month or year. If we put things off with enough regularity we may never begin. We begin to think of ourselves as ditherers and procrastinators and by this act of self-definition we give ourselves permission to be this way.

Hornbeam is the spark, the spit on the hand, the squared shoulder, ready to use when our inner drive deserts us. It helps us trust our ability to deal with the next task, and the next, and the one after. Since Bach's day it has been known as the 'Monday morning' remedy and the 'morning after' remedy. The first nickname implies the taking up of a daily task, as most people go back to work on the Monday after the weekend break. The second implies the resumption of a dull task after last night's party. And in both the word 'morning' gives a clue to the immaterial nature of the Hornbeam state. We may well be physically rested after a night's sleep – or a day spent lounging around on the beach. The problem is not physical tiredness (for which we would turn instead to Olive). Rather it is a mental fatigue, a weariness that might feel physical at the time but which is illusory. The proof of this is that our decision to begin causes it to melt away like a snowflake in summer.

> When I can't face the day I drop Hornbeam into my tea.
> Hornbeam days are over by the time I have finished drinking it.
> – Kate Anderson
>
> This remedy was particularly helpful when I worked for a short time of night duty. The first night back I would always feel tired and apprehensive at the thought of the coming shift. Hornbeam always proved very useful, enabling me to cope with the tasks ahead. – Maggie

when something goes wrong

When something goes wrong we can react in one of two main ways. The healthy way is to acknowledge what the problem is and deal with it. The unhealthy way is to make the thing that went wrong a model for other events and make assumptions based on this model. To give an example, imagine two people who have applied for a job but have been turned down. They haven't even been given an interview. We'll call them Sarah and Bob.

Sarah's response is healthy. She looks at the facts of the case so as to see what might have gone wrong. Did she explain properly why she was made redundant from her previous job? If she didn't fill out the 'other relevant information' box on the application form could she have said something there about her commitment to community causes that might have shown her energy and enthusiasm in a better light? Is her experience really relevant to the kind of job she wants? If it isn't, what can she do to get some relevant experience before filling out the next form? Or maybe she should look at applying for a different type of job altogether? Sarah tries to isolate things about the failure than can help her improve her next attempt. Her failure makes her a better-equipped job-hunter with a renewed commitment to getting where she wants to go.

Bob, on the other hand, sees the job rejection as more than a single setback. For him it is part of a pattern. From this one instance he builds up a picture of himself in which failure and disappointment are to be expected. From his point of view there is nothing to be gained from taking all the sensible steps that Sarah did. He may stop trying to get work, or continue to send in badly worded applications for jobs that wouldn't suit him. Every subsequent failure reinforces his pessimism and lack of belief in a brighter tomorrow.

We could put this a slightly different way, and say that if Sarah feels despondent when she hears she hasn't got the job, that is a feeling that she temporarily *has*. It is an emotional state outside herself, and something she can deal with. But for Bob despondency becomes a habit – either over time or all at once. By seeing his problem as a life pattern he identifies himself with the corresponding emotion. He doesn't *have* despondency. Instead he *is* despondent. And because he *is* the problem he can't step outside it and deal with it. Sarah and Bob show us the difference between *having* a bad time and deciding to *be* down, which is the difference between Gentian and Gorse.

overcome obstacles: gentian

When we are in a labyrinth every wrong turning is valuable because it teaches us more about the maze and so in the long run helps us get through it. Similarly every discouragement in our lives, every disappointment, can be an opportunity to learn. Few great successes came without a history of many failures preceding them, for without failure we learn nothing. Failure teaches us more about our situation, shows us where the way is blocked, provides an opportunity to test our strength. It reminds us to look again at what we are trying to be or do so as to check we are on the right path. Most of the time we know this in our hearts. We may grumble when things go wrong but we pick up the burden again and try a new route. Our intuition leads us right and tells us we will succeed. All we need to do is go forward and refuse to be downcast.

This is what Bach did when he first tested the Gentian remedy. Weeks tells how he looked for and found the autumn gentian in the hills beyond Ewelme, in Oxfordshire. It was July and too early to harvest the flowers, so back in Cromer later in the year he hunted for it again. But the weeks went by and he failed to find any sign of the plant. Refusing to give up, he travelled south into Kent, where he finally found it in full flower on a hillside and was able to prepare the first batch of the remedy towards the end of September, right at the end of its flowering period.

We might imagine Bach coming home with slumped shoulders after another fruitless day tramping the flat fields of Norfolk. That would be the Gentian state, one in which we doubt and feel down-hearted when things go wrong. We will take the next step and try again despite our discouragement, as indeed Bach did, but we do so with a heavier heart than we should. Taking the flower reconnects us with the blaze of our inner optimism. It helps us look for the positive side of any setback. If we didn't get the promotion we wanted we reconsider our career and may look for new opportunities elsewhere. If our troubled marriage has finally come to an end we celebrate the release as a triumph rather than thinking of it as a reverse. Gentian reminds us that there is no such thing as failure, only further opportunities to learn and move forward.

choose hope: gorse

I remember walking down to the sea in the middle of a British winter. Dabs of concentrated yellow leaped from the hedgerows, as intense as oil paint – the constant sunshine of the gorse flowers. Bach first harvested their power in 1933. The following year he wrote a letter from Cromer and told how he decided to prepare them:

> One day, feeling anxious as regards the future, as I suppose we are all liable to do at times, I was lying near the tow-path at Marlow-on-Thames, when this message came through. A message not only for myself, but for all those who are striving to help.
>
> I wrote it down as it is, and instantly noticed by my side a gorse bush in full bloom, and I thought 'How beautiful.' I had not seen it before, but then I thought of the wondrous sight of moorlands covered with the flaming bush.

The accumulated power of gorse growing in profusion along rolling hills seems to increase the life and power in each individual bud. This was the force that Bach wanted to harness in this remedy. The strength of Gorse has the power to lift people out of the rut of despair and pessimism, helping to awaken our sense of optimism and faith in life and its possibilities.

In the negative Gorse state we have given up and turned away from hope. Sometimes we have chosen pessimism, and see nothing but more failures where our friends see hope and opportunities. Sometimes other people have told us nothing can be done and we have accepted their judgement and made it our own. In either case, as we saw with the parable of Sarah and Bob, we have allowed ourselves to identify with the problem so that we can no longer look at it objectively.

The bad news is that pessimism is a self-fulfilling prophecy. The good news is that the same is true of optimism. Those of us who believe we have the ability and opportunity to do well – even if we have failed in the past – invariably do better than those of us who accept defeat and feel we can do nothing about it. This is true regardless of the innate ability we start out with. The reason is simple: optimists never give up. We try again, and again, and again. This is our secret when we triumph over the most impossible predicaments – poverty, lack of education, physical and mental illness and disability. We know that being positive is a life choice that can always be made, wherever it is we are forced to begin. We can always choose life, choose light, choose Gorse.

I was around seven or eight years old. We lived near Bordeaux. We used to spend the winter Sunday afternoons driving to the Atlantic Ocean beaches and pine forests. My parents argued all the time, near divorce, and my mother with a severe drinking problem was very hard and unloving. One Sunday afternoon walking through the pine forests, in February, the gorse bushes were blooming, painted like yellow drops on the grey curtain of the sky and sea. I remember my feelings of wonder and the warmth of the intense yellow flowers. In the despair of all these thorns there was peace, hope and warmth there for me, under the gorse bushes. – K. Cozic

3 ❀ belief

q. is belief necessary?

What if we find talk of higher selves, souls and divine purposes difficult to accept? Do we have to believe in God and an immortal soul to
benefit from the essences? Do we have to believe in reincarnation? Do
we have to be, in however broad a sense, religious?

We can answer these questions indirectly by looking at some
of the different things people believe about spiritual and personal
development. Our survey will not pretend to be more than a taster.
We will dip into just seven of the millions of different dishes offered by
different thinkers and traditions of thought – seven approaches that
have been chosen because they share fundamental values or concepts,
sometimes to a surprising degree. We will start with four beliefs from
the East before we turn to three widely differing Western views of
reality. Yet we will linger long enough to catch some of the flavours of
belief and so see how they might affect our use of flower essences.

mencius

The Chinese philosopher Mencius, who died in 289 BC, believed that
the great virtues associated with the wise and good exist in every
human being at the moment of birth. But they are only there as
potential virtues. If we don't develop them as we grow, or if we lose
sight of our essential nature, the result will be error and evil. Mencius
described life as a kind of spiritual journey that we have to take in
order to realise our innate potential. The journey involves cultivating
qi or *ch'i*, which can be understood as life or spiritual energy. The way

to cultivate this force is to behave well towards others and avoid evil acts. The truly developed individual will be strong and centred regardless of his station in life, and can be perfect as much in a hovel as in a palace. He will also be in balance with the world and with himself and will live fully all the positive emotions. While he will value reason, he will put the reasons of the heart before reason itself.

Mencius sounds like he would be at home with Bach flower remedies.

the upanishads

The *Upanishads* are a collection of Indian poetry and prose believed to have originated between 600 and 400 BC. These sacred texts teach that the way to get close to the source of all life and being and goodness (known as *Brahman*) is to understand fully the essential self or soul (the *Atman*). This is because the *Atman* is part of *Brahman*; the individual spark part of the great fire. Because we all carry this divine spark we can all develop to the point where we become perfect, a true incarnation of the ultimate principle of the universe, a selfless and pure potency and energy.

The *Upanishads* also speak of a second aspect of the self, called *purusha*. This is the ego-riddled individual personality, which must be overcome by the sage who wants to escape from illusion and find perfection.

The ancient ideas of the *Atman* and *purusha* find an echo in Edward Bach's distinction between the higher self and the personality. Bach essences and Bach's philosophical writings are increasingly well known in India today.

tagore

Some two and half millennia after the *Upanishads* were created they influenced the philosophical and religious writings of the great Indian poet Rabindranath Tagore. Accepting the impersonal ideal of *Brahman* as the ultimate reality, Tagore nevertheless maintained that this ideal energy took the form of a specific personality when it acted as a creator. This spiritual incarnation of the ultimate was the Supreme Being. The aim of the Supreme Being in creating the earth and its life was to realise the highest good, which is love of one for another. Being a single reality, *Brahman* had to create something outside itself in order to manifest this form of love.

According to Tagore, human beings at their lowest and least developed are mired in the material world and incapable of loving others. Our desire is selfish and revolves around power and greed and possession. Selfish desire hurts us because it traps us and stops us from advancing. In contrast enlightened human beings escape from self and selfishness and the snare of their own desires. Inspired by the beauty of nature, which the Supreme Being has created for just this purpose, we begin to love other humans, plants and animals, and all of nature. Once we can love the entire creation we will have expressed our soul in love for the Supreme Being, which was the aim of creation in the first place. This love finds expression through the qualities of balance and simplicity and a life lived in balance with nature: Tagore was a great planter of trees.

We have already seen how Bach's view of personal evolution stressed the need to transmute selfishness into selflessness and express this through love, and how a similar idea was expressed in psychology by Abraham Maslow's hierarchy of needs. Tagore's understanding of life echoes and confirms both.

buddhism

Long before Tagore elements of the *Upanishads* inspired another and greater teacher to create his own system of belief. Buddhism is the only great religion that doesn't spend time talking about God or claim to be divinely inspired. It is also the least bloody of sects. Its followers have never gone in for holy wars or inquisitions or forced conversion.

Instead Buddhism teaches 'the middle way', a life of tolerance and gentleness, of balance and measured action. Its founder, Siddhartha Gautama, the Buddha or enlightened one, rejected the extremes of selfish desire and spiritual martyrdom as equally unprofitable. Instead he taught how release from the endless and painful cycle of reincarnation could come through a spiral of wisdom, right action and reflection on right actions that he called 'the noble eightfold path'.

According to the Buddha, every individual is a mix of qualities: feelings, bodily form, sense perceptions, consciousness and impulses. The law of cause and effect means that a harmful moral action at any point in a person's life makes the overall spiritual state of that person a little worse, while a right action makes it a little better. The consciousness quality of any one individual survives death and is reborn into a new life. Because of this the legacy of good and bad actions carries over from one life to another. Following the eightfold path gradually improves the consciousness's position until it can escape rebirth altogether and achieve nirvana.

The ultimate aim of Buddhist thought is the greater happiness of all life. The Buddha saw individual existences as simple nodes, transitory interconnected events in the broad flow of existence. From this perspective all life is one. There is no 'I' and 'you', but instead an all-encompassing reality. When we reach nirvana we escape from the illusion of 'I' and 'you' and achieve a great and peaceful state of perfection removed from the flow of karmic law and rebirth. It may take many lifetimes to achieve this; the Buddha himself achieved enlightenment after one night of profound meditation under a tree, but only after many preparatory years of searching.

Bach also talked about the unity of all life, and we have seen how his view of individual progress included a belief in reincarnation. Like the eightfold path the essences represent a middle way of balance and patient progress on the road to enlightenment.

We turn now to the West.

physics

In *The Tao of Physics* Fritjof Capra sets out the difference between the old-fashioned mechanical physics of Isaac Newton and the new understanding based on relativity and quantum field theory. It turns out the main difference is very simple.

🌸 **In the Newtonian world** solid objects moved around in empty space.

🌸 **In the quantum world** solid objects and empty space are different aspects of the same single 'thing'.

This single 'thing' is a quantum field – energy that in certain places condenses to form the stuff that we interpret as matter. The 'thing' can be seen in different ways, and a physicist has to use different theories to explain its behaviour depending on what aspect of it she chooses to study. The aim of much of modern physics is to unify all these different theories into one. In Albert Einstein's words, the field described by a unified theory would be 'the only reality'.

As Capra points out, quantum thinking echoes those Eastern traditions that see physical reality and the self as illusions and temporary manifestations of a single underlying reality. Physics advanced so far in the twentieth century that it began to find hard proof of the East's belief in unity. We are one, even if we don't always see it that way.

psychosynthesis

From physics we move quickly to psychology, and to Dr Roberto Assagioli's system of *psychosynthesis*. Psychosynthesis is a method for achieving personal and transpersonal growth. Since its genesis in 1910 it has been among the most influential of modern approaches to psychotherapy.

At the risk of over-simplifying Assagioli's work, his model for inner development can be described in terms of an obstacle course in which four formidable barriers have to be overcome.

❧ *First*, we need to understand fully our existing personalities, which means undertaking a journey of discovery down into the unconscious and uncovering the hidden fears and conflicts that waste so much of our energy.

❧ *Second*, we have to try to control some of these conflicts and fears. This involves a process Assagioli calls disidentification. For example, if we feel afraid we usually say, 'I am afraid,' so that 'I' and 'afraid' are seen as the same thing. In other words, we identify ourselves with the feeling of fear. In order to undo this process we need to find new ways of thinking and talking about the fear. We might for example say, 'A feeling of fear is trying to overcome me.' This sets up an opposition between the emotion and the self, helping the self to resist and redirect emotional energy instead of becoming identified with it.

❧ *Third*, we have to find (or create) a centre for the self around which we can construct a true or higher self. The centre is a reason for living, a purpose and sense of upward movement that is consistent with our current status and level of development. Assagioli specifically warns against creating unrealistic or neurotic ideals that can't be achieved.

❧ *Fourth*, we begin to build up the new unified personality around its new centre by developing those qualities that currently we lack.

This is a very close description of what we do when we take flower essences: we look honestly at who we are, we objectify our emotions, we discover our purpose, we use the remedies to encourage the virtues we lack.

camus

Albert Camus was born in Algeria. He was a lover of Greek philosophers, sunbathing and sport, and still no doubt the only Nobel Prize-winner to have been a goalkeeper. He loved ordinary pleasures and ordinary people, not in some idealised or condescending way, but as an ordinary person himself. The sunlight and sea of the Mediterranean sparkle and shimmer throughout his early writing. Yet there is darkness there too. He once said he was an optimist as far as humanity was concerned but a pessimist about the human condition. His love of life only sharpened his sense of anguish at the inevitability of ageing and death.

In 1942 Camus published *Le mythe de Sisyphe*, his defining statement on the feeling of dissociation and meaninglessness that he called *the absurd*. In Greek legend Sisyphus was a mortal man in constant rebellion against the gods. Alive, he betrayed Jupiter and imprisoned Death. Dead, he persuaded Pluto to allow him one more short stay on earth then refused to return to Hades when his time was up. Mercury had to seize him and drag him back to the underworld. As a punishment for his transgressions the gods condemned Sisyphus to push a heavy rock up a mountain for all eternity. Every time he got the rock to the top it would roll back down by itself. Sisyphus had to walk back down to the bottom of the mountain and start again.

Camus saw in the punishment of Sisyphus a symbol of the endless struggle of mortal existence, reduced and made meaningless by the fact of death. Because there is no aim to the universe, he said, our every action is as empty as Sisyphus rolling his stone up the mountain. The central problem of *Le mythe de Sisyphe* was therefore the problem of suicide. In other words, having rejected belief in God and appalled at the idea of a meaningless life, why should Camus not kill himself now? He loved life too much to *want* to kill himself, but believing in the absurd he faced the problem of finding a philosophical justification for his gut instinct to go on living. What rational reason was there to continue?

Camus based his moral philosophy on courage, honesty and a desire for unity with the universe or (since he believed that was almost certainly not possible) unity at least with the rest of humanity. He did not believe in God or any more-than-human reality that might offer hope or salvation or transcendent meaning. Instead he described 'a sort of difficult march towards a saintliness of negation [and] the pure man'. We have to develop, he said, in order to make a meaning. He condemned judicial killing on the grounds that killing someone removed that person's chance of becoming perfect. He rejected those political systems that demand misery today as the price for some imaginary future, and instead supported the right of each individual to grow freely and find his own path. He talked about humanity's task being the creation of God, and that the only way to create God was to *become* God. He wrote that if there was a soul it wasn't something that was already created, but something that we create in living our lives. Living, for Camus, is a long and tortured birth pang for the soul.

In a notebook entry written in the spring of 1943 Camus made a distinction between *evidential* philosophy, in other words a philosophy based on the perceived facts, and *preferred* philosophy, which is what one aspires towards. His evidential philosophy was the absurd and the impossibility of living in it. But his preferred philosophy upheld the possibility of fulfilment and of a just and harmonious balance between spirit and world. In his notebooks Camus dismissed his preferred philosophy in the name of a determined refusal to corrupt the facts as he saw them. But *Le mythe de Sisyphe* itself ends with an astonishing leap of faith that inclines us to believe that he gave more weight than he thought to his preference. For in the end Sisyphus's struggle to roll the stone to the top of the mountain was not meaningless. It contained, Camus tells us, the elements of effort and aspiration that are enough to make Sisyphus – incredibly, wonderfully – happy.

parallels

We can see from this that Camus was far from being a hard-nosed and complacent atheist. Instead he was the most troubled and haunted of twentieth-century thinkers, with a genuine desire to speak for and enunciate the psychological and philosophical anguish of those who lived in the time of the Holocaust and the Gulag. He always left room for doubt and had none of the arrogance of other more systematic thinkers. 'At the limit of intelligence,' he wrote, 'we know for sure that there is some truth in all theory.'

This is real wisdom. And if we turn back to Bach's view of humanity and the universe and compare them with the other belief systems we have looked at, we can see that not only is there some truth in all of them, but that often the truths are the same.

- ✿ **Like Mencius**, Bach believed we should all develop our better qualities, keep contact with our innermost nature and express the positive emotions of love and charity and solidarity. Both believed that we should be true to our personal path in life, whether rich or poor, live without envy and try to do good to others. Both believed that our essential inner balance and unity should be reflected in a state of balance with other people and with the universe.
- ✿ **Like the *Upanishads***, Bach's writings deal with the need to understand our essential selves so as fully to express the divinity within us. Bach echoes the sacred texts when he roots the egoistic personality in the material world and contrasts it with the more spiritual and more essentially real higher self.
- ✿ **Like Tagore**, Bach equated nature with goodness and saw the love of plants and animals as a divine path leading towards a more balanced and spiritual life. Both talk of the transmuting of selfishness into selflessness and of the need to turn away from possessions and greed and towards freedom and love of others.

❁ **Like Buddha**, Bach stressed balance and condemned the kind of spiritual extremism that seeks perfection through pain and martyrdom. Both saw how wisdom might only come after many lifetimes of struggle and striving. Both stressed the harm that cruelty did to the cruel, greed to the greedy, selfishness to the selfish. Both stressed the fundamental unity of all life.

❁ **Like today's physicists**, Bach believed in the ultimate interconnectedness of everything in the universe. He would have understood the emerging science of ecology and its picture of life as a magical pattern of interdependence in which every thread in the tapestry is linked to every other.

❁ **Like Assagioli**, Bach saw the need to uncover hidden emotions working from the outside in. Both speak of redirecting emotional energy and encouraging its positive manifestation rather than trying to suppress or repress the negative. Both speak of bringing the personality into line with a higher conception of the self and of the need to encourage and reinforce those positive virtues that are not yet fully developed.

❁ **Like Camus**, Bach believed that people grow better if they concentrate on their qualities rather than thinking of their failings. Both believed that the more profound virtue lay in balancing emotions rather than in suppressing them. Both believed in the individual's right to grow and find perfection in his own individual way. Both believed in the ideal of unity and condemned actions that hurt other people or that interfere with the freedom of others.

In all these traditions enlightenment comes when we understand our relationships with each other and with existence in general. Indeed, personal and spiritual growth and a greater awareness of interconnectedness are the same thing. True self-development does not equal selfishness, as its critics claim — rather it transcends the self and includes the universe. Without awareness of its connection with the universe the personality might well take self-expression to mean the unbridled fulfilment of its narrow desires. But awareness of unity acts as a check. Any action that damages another or destroys beauty or in any other way breaks us off from our roots is seen to be wrong in and of itself. Wrong actions separate us from the whole. We are diminished when we do things out of petty self-interest, and growth means getting bigger, not smaller. If Camus is right and we need to become God we will have to grow big enough to accept and welcome and love everything. This means moving so far away from our everyday concerns that we annihilate the narrow self. In Bach's words:

> [T]he cause of all our troubles is self and separateness, and this vanishes as soon as love and the knowledge of the great Unity become part of our natures. ... [R]eal love must be infinitely above our ordinary comprehension, something tremendous, the utter forgetfulness of self, the losing of the individuality in the unity, the absorption of the personality in the whole.

a. is belief necessary?

The antique worlds of Greece and Rome embraced religious tolerance and accepted the cross-fertilisation of disparate beliefs. Like many modern spiritual thinkers and more progressive elements in the organised religions, Bach goes back to this ancient tradition and sees value in different approaches to spirituality. He thought of himself as a Christian, but still spoke with respect of other belief systems and at times borrowed from them. And his model for how evolution takes place – bringing the personality into line with the needs of an already perfected higher self – is not orthodox Christianity. Nor is belief in reincarnation.

When we analyse world religions and humanist philosophies we find that they all contain the same basic human aspirations towards growth, purity, unity and connectedness. All talk about our place in the world and about how we can be better, and that of course is what the essences are about. We have the liberty to be eclectic, just as Bach was, and understand the concepts in his philosophical writings as direct truth or as a metaphor for any other belief system that promotes ethical, spiritual or personal growth and development. When Bach talks of the higher self and the need to follow its commands we can understand this as an expression of our need to develop towards something greater and higher and more aware than we are now. Whether we call that something higher self, soul, spirit, God, essential self, *Atman*, potential virtue, nature, Supreme Being, enlightenment, unity, nirvana, true self, ideal self, pure man or anything else is less important than the aspiration to grow from where we are and find a way to be more of what we can be. We can't expect to know what the top of the mountain *really* looks like until we reach it. We will never reach it unless we make up our minds to begin the climb.

Bach always insisted on people's right to make their own choices so it is fitting that the philosophy behind remedy use should not be exclusive. Flower essences put the power of healing and self-knowledge into our hands irrespective of our religious and philosophical and cultural beliefs. Indeed there is a very real sense in which we should put our theories aside when using the remedies. 'They who will obtain the greatest benefit from this God-sent Gift,' wrote Dr Bach shortly before he died, 'will be those who keep it pure as it is; free from science, free from theories, for everything in Nature is simple.' So not only can Buddhists, Christians, Hindus, humanists, atheists and others all use the remedies, but we can all use them in the same way: selecting them according to how we feel, taking them when we need to, and as a result helping ourselves to develop and grow.

We asked several questions at the start of this chapter. What if we find all this talk of higher selves, souls and divine purposes difficult to accept? Does one have to believe in God and an immortal soul to benefit from the remedies? Does one have to believe in reincarnation? Does one have to be, in however broad a sense, religious?

The answer to these questions is, no, we don't have to believe in this or that religious concept, but, yes, we do have to believe in one thing, namely *the possibility of being better than we are*. The philosophy of the thirty-eight flowers is truly ecumenical. Anybody of any faith can embrace it and put it to good use because, as Hermia Brockway of the Japanese organisation Bach Holistic Kenkyukai points out, it is always aimed at our spiritual betterment. 'The philosophical background to the remedies is extremely positive,' she says. 'It's an ideal and uplifting frame of reference spelling out that it is our birthright to find happiness.' This is the essential. The rest we can leave to whichever god we find.

a personal postscript

One reader of an early draft of this chapter said that this was the part where the author disappeared. Perhaps I should put myself back in, she suggested, because it seemed odd that I should be so suddenly absent. I mulled this over. Maybe, I thought, the disappearance of 'I' is right in a chapter that talks about the need to transcend the self. The pronoun 'we' appears a lot, not 'I', and so it should. Further thought brought a different slant on things, and a new and more uncomfortable possibility. Perhaps I took myself out of this chapter because I am in fact a person who finds it difficult to talk about souls and divine purposes. When teaching and writing in the past I have always been most at home with the practicalities of remedy use – the kitchen cabinet was more comfortable to me than the sacred grove – so maybe I was just dodging a challenge.

This felt true, but only up to a point. I love and have always loved sacred groves – and old churches, and stone circles, and the sea – everything that smacks of eternity and might in some way transcend the physical facts of birth and copulation and death. So why did I write myself out of this chapter? What was it in particular that made me uncomfortable?

I think the answer might be this: that I don't myself believe in the Christian conception of a personal God. Many of Bach's writings presuppose this belief, which is certainly one that he held himself. In working at the Bach Centre and in supporting and promoting his system of remedies to the best of my ability, and in particular in helping others who *do* believe in a personal God to see how his work is valid for them, I have got into the habit of leaving my own beliefs to one side. Which is why, even in a chapter that explicitly says that the remedies are useful regardless of what we believe, the personal 'I' once more stepped aside as soon as a personal God became central to the discussion. And because I think this is a bad habit that I have fallen into – Bach was clear that we should state our truths in a straightforward way and above all be ourselves – I am taking my reader's advice and stepping back in.

So what do I personally believe? This chapter shows that the question is irrelevant in so far as it has no effect on how you and I use remedies. We can agree to differ and still work with and learn from each other. But for the record let me say that I love Camus more than any other single thinker mentioned here, although I disagree with him on one central point. Camus felt with others of his time that consciousness – the essence of what it is to be human – was irrevocably split off from the material world and from nature. I think that is wrong. Consciousness is as natural as light and air. And far from being split, everything in nature connects. Like Camus, I'm inclined to believe that there is no individual creator God in our human past. But all of us have godlike qualities in us, because the idea of 'God' – like Bach's idea of the higher self – can be understood as a goal, something towards which we aim, something of which we are capable if we can only move up the pyramid and reach the level of self-actualisation where we transcend ourselves and fully see and feel our connection with each other and with the universe. So despite the absence of a creator God in the past there may well be something Godlike in our human future. And with that thought I retire and resume my story.

iii ❀ the swayed heart

How many folk can you number amongst your friends or relations who are free? How many are there who are not bound or influenced or controlled by some other human being? How many are there who could say, that day by day, month by month, and year by year, 'I obey only the dictates of my soul, unmoved by the influence of other people?'
– Edward Bach

four remedies for the swayed heart

We all have our own path in life. To walk that path successfully we sometimes need to rise above circumstances and break old habits. Other times opinions and ideas hold us back – other people's or our own – and we need to shake them off so as to grow. The four essences in this section help us to do this. They were described by Bach as being for people who are especially subject to influences and ideas.

❀ **Agrimony** lets us understand our dark side and our worries and reintegrate them into the whole personality. The Agrimony person is over-sensitive to her negative thoughts and so tries to keep the surface of life unruffled. She adopts a false smile that hides problems instead of dealing with them.

❀ The particular strength of **Centaury** lies in serving and helping. This leaves her open to abuse by more ruthless personalities, so that she can end up neglecting her own needs completely.

❀ **Walnut** tries to move ahead but finds that her own past or other people's opinions and ideas stop her from changing and developing. She needs to disregard past events and present climates of opinion and follow her inner voice if she knows it is right.

🌸 **Holly** is attacked by violent, spiteful thoughts about other people. There might be suspicion verging on paranoia, hate, envy or a desire to pay somebody back for some real or imagined wrong. The remedy can help her to rise above these negative thoughts and move into a space from which she can return love for hate.

the great clown

Joseph Grimaldi was a comic singer, acrobat and actor. He was born in London in 1779. His family, who came originally from Italy, were already established on the London stage, and the young Grimaldi appeared as an infant dancer at the Drury Lane Theatre before his second birthday. A year later he made his debut on the stage at Sadler's Wells, and by the time he was in his early twenties he was the best-known clown in England. His use of costume influenced every clown who came after him. The habit of calling clowns 'Joey' is a reminder of his celebrity.

Grimaldi was such a great comedian that doctors would send their depressed patients to see him instead of giving them drugs. On one occasion in the 1820s an especially unhappy man consulted a doctor in great secrecy about his depression. 'Nothing lifts it,' he said, 'life is a torture to me and I don't know how I can face it any more.'

The doctor gave the same answer he gave to all his patients. 'The great clown Grimaldi is playing at Sadler's Wells. Go to see him. Nobody who sees Grimaldi can remain down for long.'

'But, Doctor,' said the man, 'I am Grimaldi.'

Overwork, ill-health and exhaustion forced Joseph Grimaldi to retire from the stage in 1828. He died in 1837.

know yourself: agrimony

From time to time we all pretend to feel better than we do. Perhaps it's a legacy of our upbringing when we were told to stop crying, not make a fuss, put on a brave face, smile through our tears. Unfortunately the people saying these things were probably thinking of their own peace of mind more than of ours. Putting barriers up around painful feelings doesn't solve them. All it does is push them down into fertile soil. The pain festers in closed parts of our minds ready to re-emerge when our guard is down, when we are alone with our thoughts, trying to relax, lying awake in bed. The psychologist Robert Holden goes so far as to claim that ninety per cent of pain is actually caused by the effort of keeping pain secret.

Barriers aren't selective. If we shut away our worries behind a big smiley front that same big smiley front will cut us off from other feelings as well. We need to be in touch with all our emotions if we want to feel genuine happiness, confidence, courage and joy. If we avoid solitude we will never appreciate real friendship. If we make small jokes of everything we will never aspire to that great-hearted humour that loves, grieves and laughs all at once. If we refuse the depths we will stay shallow. We need to acknowledge the pain in the dark half of our hearts because that is where we will find the qualities we need to overcome pain and gain true peace. As the poet David Whyte puts it, 'wanting soul life without the dark, warming intelligence of personal doubt is like expecting an egg without the brooding heat of the mother hen.'

In the negative Agrimony state we turn away from the brooding heat and the heart of darkness. Healing humour becomes a mask and a barrier. We wear a bright smile and a brave face, while underneath we suffer torture and an unquiet spirit. Being alone is a trial to us because we find it harder to hide. We may use drink or drugs, or seek out crowds, excitement and bright lights as a relief from our pain and a way of keeping the grin fixed in place. We may suffer from insomnia as our tortured thoughts return to us in the small hours before dawn.

The Agrimony essence gives us the ability to experience the dark and come through it enriched. It takes away pretence and concealment and magnifies humour to the status of a philosophy. It allows us to be

I feel Agrimony has helped me a lot. I'm not so eager to keep everybody happy and much as I hate arguments I'm standing my ground regardless of the discomfort. I have been able to cry and remove the brave face. – Linda Lewcock

I started to feel different. Initially, I admit, these differences didn't seem pleasant. But as time moved on I became aware that it was a process I had to go through in order to feel better. Due to keeping my true feelings inside and outwardly always pretending I was fine I wasn't always aware of the sort of things I had stored away inside me. I had played the part for so long I wasn't aware it was an act. Thank you, for one, Agrimony. – Avril Harvey

When I first read the description of Agrimony I instantly related to it. It helped me take a leap in self-awareness as I began to look more honestly at my hidden pains and sorrows, and realise what avoidance tactics I had been using. I started to see that alcohol was not a true friend. I am still not one to pour my heart out, but I feel Agrimony helped me to express my true feelings more easily. – Michael Hillier

I practised t'ai chi with a friend. One day she gave me some feedback about how she saw me. She felt I was an Agrimony type person as I always seemed cheerful and happy despite the difficult situations I was in and the hard times I was going through. I don't think anyone had been so frank and honest with me before in such a kind and giving way. She gave me a bottle of Agrimony and suggested I try it. Not only did it open me up more to talk about myself but it also inspired me to look at my behaviour patterns more deeply and seek a life of greater quality. – Elaine Arthey

THE SWAYED HEART ❀ 71

fully aware of the dark side yet still take joy in life. Agrimony is always the peace-maker and the peace-lover, able to find agreement between opposites and alive to the possibility of compromise and social cohesion. She is always a good companion among good companions, who believes that if we work together with love and laughter we will find a way through our difficulties. But she can let her pain out and share it honestly with others. In this way she finds the single most effective way of reducing it.

serve yourself: centaury

I am weak, yes, I know I am weak, but why? Because I have learnt to hate strength and power and dominion, and if I do err a little on the weakness side, forgive me, because it is only a reaction to the hatred of hurting others, and I shall soon learn to understand how to find the balance when I neither hurt nor am hurting. But just for the moment I would rather that I suffered than that I caused one moment's pain to my brother.

So be very patient with your little Centaury, she is weak, I know, but it is a weakness on the right side, and I shall soon grow bigger and stronger and more beautiful until you will all admire me because of the strength I shall bring to you.

Edward Bach

When we talk about remedies and about personality characteristics we find it useful sometimes to make broad distinctions. These character traits are introvert, those are extrovert; these are active, those passive; these short-term, those long-term. Classifying people and essences helps us think about emotions in a structured way. But our clearly divided categories are never exact matches to the world, for in nature all opposites eventually meet. This is especially true of the opposition between strong and weak that points to the difference between those who make a noise and take charge (remedies would include Vervain, Vine, Chicory) and those who are quiet and taken charge of (Larch, Mimulus and, above all, Centaury). At some level we all are and must be strong.

About eighteen of the remedy plants grow in the garden at the Bach Centre. The exact number varies from year to year, as the plants self-seed where they please. When the flowering times come we have to search for some of them. In particular the early growth of centaury is often hard to spot in the tangle of greenery. But a couple of years ago one particular plant couldn't be missed. It forced its way up through the cracks in one of the paths. We don't usually take special care of the remedy plants in the garden because they have to grow wild, but we made an exception for this one and roped it off in case any visitors trod on it before the flowers came.

The positive qualities of Centaury are the positive characteristics of that plant: self-reliance, independence and a determination to grow its own way. This doughty weed eventually supplied flowers for that year's batch of remedy, so we might add a further quality to the list: a desire to help others and to serve. Indeed, this is the key to Centaury because it shows the direction that she takes in the negative state. Bach defines love somewhere as 'service combined with wisdom'. In the negative Centaury state the wisdom has gone. A desire to help others becomes the inability to refuse others, and from a free helper we turn into a slave.

The 'typical' Centaury is the dutiful daughter who takes care of her ageing father. Her brothers and sisters are happy to leave the job to her, the father relies more and more on her help, and she herself finds it easier to deny herself than deny others. So she misses out on social events, work and study opportunities. Later she misses out on romance and the chance to have children of her own. Her energy and essence – all the things she could have achieved and the directions in which she could have developed – go to feed the flame of somebody else's life. Bach had harsh words for parents who try to push their children into this lamentable state. 'It is impossible to calculate the thousands of hindered lives,' he wrote, 'the myriads of missed opportunities, the sorrow and the suffering so caused, the countless number of children who from a sense of duty have perhaps for years waited upon an invalid when the only malady the parent has known has been the greed of attention.'

This may seem hard on our loved ones: what if the need is real and we are the only available carer? But even here the message repays hearing. Always providing immediate service is by no means the best way to help others. If a doting mother bails her son out of every financial problem he will never learn to stand on his own feet. If a dutiful daughter accepts her enslavement she encourages her father's slide into dependence and makes possible the self-interested blindness of his family and neighbours and society itself. A measure of freedom and independence helps the people we love; an inability to refuse hurts everybody. However loving and helpful we are and however great the needs of others our higher duty is to leave ourselves and them space and time to go different ways.

If we are true Centaury types we will want to help others. A vocation to serve will bring us the sense of rightness and fulfilment that is its own intrinsic value, and will influence all our decisions in life. But before we turn down this road we need to be sure that what we take for a divine mission is not in fact our weakness in the face of somebody else's power. Saying 'yes' in freedom is very different from not being able to say 'no', and learning to say 'no' is part of defining the self, part of growing up, something we must all do before we can fully engage in the world. Having learned this lesson, the positive Centaury can serve when she chooses to, and serve wisely, and refuse to serve if that is the right thing for her or the other person. She is in contact with her inner sense of direction and will listen to the whisper of that voice rather than the stern commands of other earth-bound personalities. And like our fragile path-grown plant she will find her way up to the light in her own way and where she chooses, with such strength that nothing will stop her.

Centaury had an amazing effect. It was as if I became an observer, viewing what others were doing to me and my own reactions. I realised I didn't need to accept this behaviour and I was able to step aside and away from the situation. I no longer allow myself to be put upon or demeaned in any way. – Sylvia Rymer-Lawes

I was working in a chemist's shop and my boss didn't want to let me go. With Centaury I managed to tell him that I wanted to leave. It came out in a very gentle way and the parting was not in the least painful or acrimonious. It gave me leave to feel pleased with myself and it also gave my confidence a boost. – Sylvia Spence

I was draining myself of energy by never saying 'no' to anyone, and Centaury was prescribed. Always a caring person, I had not realised that it was having an adverse effect on me. – Pamela Higginson

At the moment I am treating myself with the Centaury remedy to help me give more consideration to myself and my needs. You notice the difference in a subtle way. When faced with a difficult situation you suddenly find yourself thinking and acting more positively and then you stop and say to yourself, 'Gosh, is this me?' Then you remember that you are taking the remedy and you say to yourself, 'Is this the remedy? It must be, this proves it works, what a wonderful treatment.' – Sheila Bennett

old habits die hard

Imagine a flat country. When it rains the drops collect and flow from one low point to another. At first there are many trickles of water stroking the earth in all directions, but the lowest parts attract the most trickles and so get worn away first. Over time channels appear. As water runs to a channel it carries earth down to be swept away, and so a shallow valley forms to either side. The deeper the channel the wider the valley and so the more likely it is that rain falling anywhere nearby will end up flowing through it. The deeper and wider channels deepen further into river beds. More and more of the minor flows turn into tributaries of the rivers, which become deep and permanent scars leading to the sea.

Our every action and thought triggers a pattern of connections in the brain. Like a trickle of water over flat land, most thoughts come and go and leave no trace. But we repeat some of them and so activate the same pattern again. If we fire the pattern enough times we stamp synaptic sequences into the brain and they fix, form virtual watercourses into which any nearby floating thought is likely to fall. Habits are streams, old habits rivers, and our electric thoughts run towards these paths of least resistance. This is why breaking habits and adjusting to change can be so difficult. Changing a habit means changing the course of a river and getting the charge of thought to follow a new track.

If we only had to re-route the rivers in one country that would be bad enough. Dealing with other people makes change even harder. Our friends and family create pictures of who we are and what we do, channels in their own minds, and these too fix us in position. 'It won't last,' they say in a comfortable voice when they notice our efforts to change our lives. 'He's always the same.' We will only convince our friends when we move so insistently away from who we were that they can no longer make us fit into the old bed. Until then their assumptions will be a hand on our elbow guiding us back into our old place. And some will resist our efforts to change for more personal reasons. Changing their view of us would force them to change their view of themselves. We see this happen when we grow into adulthood. To our parents we remain children because they have defined themselves as parents. Allowing us to grow up means they have to change too, and find new things to do with their lives. They may not want to. Addicts see a similar pattern. When an alcoholic tells his drinking buddies that he has to stop the booze their first reaction is often to deny there's a problem. Accepting that a friend is an alcoholic – especially one they drink with every day – means too great a challenge to their own self-image.

Finally, our cultural background also tends to fix us in place. We share the assumptions of our society. Going a different way, even if we feel it is right, even if we have thought things through properly, may mean defying our culture's definition of common sense. Not all of us have faith enough to do this, or at least not without help. Yet if the way we want to change is right for us – even if it would be wrong for every other person who has lived since the world began – we need to find the will to go through with it. Otherwise we risk stopping our development. We risk stagnation as the unchallenged river deepens to a still and landlocked sea.

grow your way: walnut

Farmers often planted walnut trees near grazing land because insects stayed away from them, giving livestock a refuge from summer flies and midges. The name itself comes from the Old English word *wealh*, meaning foreign, and reflects the fact that the walnut tree came originally from Persia. A *wealh* nut is a foreign nut, yet the walnut tree has naturalised in Britain and Europe and has managed to thrive despite the different climate.

The Walnut flower helps us to grow like the tree, in our own way, whether we are living in soil foreign to us or struggling against our upbringing or the opinions of others. It is helpful at all times of change, including the normal changes associated with different stages of life: weaning, teething, starting school, changing jobs, getting married and so on. With the help of Walnut we can adjust more quickly to new surroundings and new demands, while all the time remaining true to ourselves. Walnut is both an agent of (right) change, then, and a protection against the bites and buzzes of (wrong) change. And what is right or wrong for us is of course what is right or wrong for our higher selves, not what is right or wrong for society or our friends or parents or partners. When we try to be different and old habits or our current situation hold us back Walnut helps sever the links. Bach called it 'a great spell-breaker, both of things of the past commonly called heredity, and circumstances of the present'.

We can see negative and positive Walnut states in the life of the pianist and composer Emmanuel Chabrier. Born in 1841, Chabrier was a talented amateur musician from an early age but nevertheless allowed his father to persuade him to study law and prepare for a career in public administration. After his studies ended Chabrier worked at the French Ministry of the Interior for eighteen years. Music was no more than a serious hobby. Here is the negative Walnut: allowing the opinions of others to turn us aside from what we want.

The crisis for Chabrier came when he attended a performance of Richard Wagner's *Tristan und Isolde* in 1879. Normally a sociable and light-hearted man, Chabrier was profoundly affected by Wagner's dramatic and grandiose music. Immediately after the performance he shut himself away to try to come to terms with the experience. When he emerged from his cocoon it was with the conviction that music was his true calling. The following year he left his job and devoted himself to it full time.

Chabrier remained a champion of Wagner's music all his life. But with few exceptions – the intense gloom of the opera *Gwendoline* is one – he remained true to his own musical genius, which was for light opera and joyous piano and orchestral pieces full of good humour, ironic wit and lightly worn sensibility. (According to legend, the musicians rehearsing for the first performance of his *Joyeuse Marche* laughed out loud at the sheer delight of playing the music.) And this of course is the positive Walnut: taking the good out of an influence but not being deflected by it; moving forward in our own way and marching, joyously, to the beat of our own drum.

In my yoga classes I found myself becoming increasingly sensitive to the sometimes depressing and negative feelings emanating from students. Practising yoga postures helps to release these feelings and as a teacher I was very aware of what was happening. Walnut helped me cope with this and retain my detachment. – Cath Harper

After separating from my partner, changing careers and dealing with issues I had suppressed for years, I was trying to pull myself out of a depression. The first remedy I bought was Walnut. I took it for six weeks, at the end of which time I decided to commit myself to another relationship and stopped drinking alcohol, something that had been a vital crutch for many years. It wasn't until years later that I realised the Walnut had helped me to release the addiction. – Gillian Smith

Although the decision to take early retirement had been mine and I was relieved in many ways to be free there were aspects of the job I loved and I knew I would miss. Walnut helped me to adapt. – E.M.

I was trying to distance myself from a very domineering and rather manipulative friend who had become intrusive. Somebody suggested I take Walnut. A few days later I noticed that the large tree in our neighbour's garden is, in fact, a Walnut. I remember feeling profoundly moved at this discovery. Taking the remedy helped me to distance myself from this person and enjoy a sense of freedom. – Angela

On Christmas Day 1989 I had an accident at work and sustained a back injury which resulted in six months' incapacity and the beginning of many changes in my life. Taking the remedy helped me focus on myself and how I was feeling and coping with day-to-day life. I felt in control and in a position to steer my life in the direction I wanted to go. I came to realise that this 'accident' was no accident, but a turning point in my life which opened up so many things for me. – Janet Duffill

I had become over-sensitive to my environment and I was swayed by the opinions of others when not listening to my inner guidance. This was the remedy I took when moving houses several times. Walnut helped me to be less stressed, tired and sensitive to the scattered energies when I was amongst crowds and city life. – Rosemary Barry

Finding myself single again in mid-life, after being married for a long time, was quite a change. I felt as if the whole world had turned upside down. I had to make all the decisions on my own and be the sole provider after not having gone to work for many years. Walnut was a favourite in helping me adjust to my new life. – Julia

a trusting heart

In a fine reflection of spiritual reality, hostility does more physical damage to the heart than any other kind of negative emotion, including anxiety, stress and hurry sickness. In one study, medical students with high hostility ratings were seven times more likely to die before fifty than their less hostile colleagues. In another, taking steps to reduce hostility by weeding out aggressive and suspicious thought patterns helped to reduce the incidence of second heart attacks among recovering patients. One researcher, Dr Redford Williams of Duke University, summed up his findings to Daniel Goleman: 'The antidote to hostility is to develop a more trusting heart.'

One obvious way to develop a trusting heart is to tell ourselves that people are not out to get us, and try to see things from their point of view. The driver who slows down suddenly and holds us up doesn't know that we are in a hurry. She may be lost or trying to deal with a crying child. The friend who fails to say something nice about our new haircut or clothes is not trying to belittle or criticise. She may have some trouble on her mind that we know nothing about. Understanding the point of view of others, giving them the benefit of the doubt and remembering times when we have been in the same position: these ways of seeing put brakes on the runaway train of self-righteousness. If we can do this as soon as we begin to feel our aggression rising that's great; more usually we need to cool down first, which is why psychologists advise hostile people to get away from the other person and do something that distracts their minds from their anger. The distraction can be exercise, relaxation, yoga, watching TV – anything that slows the body down. Having spent at least twenty minutes away from the anger we can go back to the situation and use our understanding and openness to deal with it in a constructive way.

Still, the obstacles are formidable. Once we decide to hate we can always find reasons to feed our hatred. The channels of suspicion run deep at the sectarian poles of Northern Ireland, and we see similar patterns in the self-righteous hostility of racist politicians and football hooligans. Society itself excuses revenge with an endless series of stories in the cinema and on TV. 'Don't get mad, get even' seems to be an accepted and acceptable way of life. And it feels good. Hate is a powerful and exciting emotion full of energy and blood and a fierce glee. Perhaps this is the real reason it escapes our control so easily.

choose love: holly

Folklore has always considered holly a sacred plant and a guardian against evil spirits and black magic. The red berries link it to life's blood, and the tree itself is so full of life that it stays green and glossy all year round. But its main symbolic resonance today comes from Christian iconography, in which the prickles remind us of the crown of thorns, and the scarlet berries stand for the blood shed to save humanity from sin. Holly is a symbol of love so absolute that it abandons the self and selfish desire. Yet at the same time the plant expresses the opposite of love – revenge, cruelty and the infliction of pain – as we find when we try to make the remedy and get caught by the prickly leaves.

As a flower remedy Holly expresses the same movement from hostility to love. In the negative state we distrust others and wish them ill. We would like to get our own back, to hurt them the way they (seem to be) hurting us. Hatred, envy, jealousy, suspicion and vengefulness are all negative Holly states. By contrast we send out loving and generous thoughts in the positive state and return good for evil. (The image of Jesus turning the other cheek comes to mind.) Holly reminds us that we are valuable and valued, loveable and loved, so that instead of being suspicious of other people we begin to see their likeness to ourselves and so assume their motives are as good as our own. Holly connects us with the fundamental unity in the universe. There can be no hatred of others when we and they are part of the same whole.

A word of warning applies to Holly. People with a nodding acquaintance with the Bach system sometimes use it as if it were the single and only remedy for anger or, just as misleading, prescribe it on the basis of its positive aspiration towards love instead of looking to see if the negative Holly state is actually present. Any of us who seem a bit harsh or rigid or snappy or selfish can end up being given Holly 'to increase our love aspect' or 'help us love ourselves' or 'open up our heart to the universe'. Though well meant, selections like these are often useless because the people making them fail to consider more appropriate essences. Anger is only a surface emotion; to select remedies for it we need to look for its underlying cause. Holly helps when the cause turns out to be hatred, spite, suspicion or envy.

Three years after my divorce I needed to release the anger inside me against my ex and against men in general. My reaction to Holly was both physical and mental, and actually amazed me. It opened me up. First I felt a definite release of tension and pressure, then I found that I was more relaxed around people of both sexes. I began to feel a flow of love from me towards others and by the end of six weeks I felt much freer within myself. – Flor Tavor

A close friend found a new girlfriend who was jealous of our friendship. My husband and I had helped him through some very difficult times and suddenly he didn't want to be with us any more. I felt betrayed and angry, and my hatred toward my ex-friend was more powerful than anything I had ever felt in my life. It was at this time that I read an article on Bach flower remedies. I felt rather cynical, but from the brief outline I felt Holly was appropriate. Within weeks my feelings had sub-sided. This was fascinating to me: as a scientist I was driven by logic, so when something worked I wanted to know the reason behind it. – Danielle

I think in terms of the remedies, using their names as symbols for the attitudes and states of mind they refer to, like having a new language. It is easier and more objective to say 'I need Holly' than to be feeling 'I hate him and I want with all my hatred to destroy him', but only acknowledging half of the feeling and finding it difficult to get to grips with resolving it. – Charles Callis

4 ❀ simplicity

bach's path

The story of Edward Bach's life provides an example of somebody finding his path early on and following it to the end regardless of every consideration, including money, status and family relationships. Even apparent detours were part of the path, although he couldn't have seen this at the time. For example, when he left school aged sixteen he didn't want to ask his father to pay for him to study medicine and so started work at the family brass foundry in Birmingham. This wrong turning gave him an understanding of the lives of working people and allowed him to see illness from their point of view. For people paid by the hour or by the day sickness meant loss of income and no bread on the family table, so that the fear of falling ill was a health problem in its own right. Later on this insight helped him move towards a new way of treating his patients.

Eventually Bach did tell his father about his wish to study medicine. His father agreed to support him through medical school. Perhaps his son's obvious lack of business sense eased the parental decision. Bach would return from client meetings with full order books, but he was unable to argue for realistic prices and the firm couldn't make any money out of the deals he made.

illness and recovery

Bach studied at Birmingham University for a time then went to finish his medical training at University College Hospital in London. He remained in London for many years, taking on various roles as researcher, consultant, pathologist and bacteriologist, often doing two or three jobs at once. He became a workaholic and spent every moment in his laboratory or on the wards. Nora Weeks points out the irony in this lover of country walks and open spaces channelling all his energies into lamp-lit rooms and hospital corridors.

> He would even avoid the London parks, fearing that the call of Nature would prove too strong for him and distract him from his work which, it seemed to him, must for the moment lie where he had the opportunity to study many patients, thinking that only in the hospital wards and laboratories would he find out how truly to relieve the sufferings of those patients. He did not know then that the love of Nature which he was doing his best to stifle was, in the end, to guide him in his search, and that the wild flowers held in their petals a far greater power of healing than any remedy prepared in the laboratory by scientific methods.

As so often happens when we try too hard Bach's efforts held him back. The strain of overwork and the lack of fresh air led to breakdowns in health. The most serious came in July 1917 when he haemorrhaged and collapsed. Still unconscious, he was taken directly to an operating theatre where colleagues from University College Hospital removed a cancerous growth. When he came round his doctors had bad news for him. The cancer was likely to spread and he could expect to live no more than three months.

Bach now proved the wisdom of William Blake's dictum, that a fool can become wise if he will only persist in his folly. As soon as he was able to walk he left his bed and went back to his research. He was determined to use the little time that he had left as best he could and make if possible some lasting contribution to humanity. The sight of the lamp burning in his window became so familiar that the hospital staff nicknamed his laboratory 'the light that never goes out'. He immersed himself in work so that it became all-consuming and effort-less. He hardly noticed the weeks roll by until, the three month dead-line long past, he realised that he had recovered his strength and was in better health than he had been for years. As Weeks says:

> This made him pause to consider the reason of his marvellous recovery, of his return to life, as it were; and he came to the conclusion that an absorbing interest, a great love, a definite purpose in life was the deciding factor of man's happiness on earth, and was indeed the incentive which had carried him through his difficulties and had helped him in the regaining of his own health.

Bach seems to have entered that state of heightened focus and ability that psychologists call *flow*. As we will see further on in *Bloom*, flow is a state of balance and wholeness. By persisting in his folly, single-mindedly and with all his heart, Bach achieved again the balance he had lost.

development

We can gauge Bach's spiritual development over the course of his life by looking at the way his intuitive powers grew. When he was an orthodox researcher using clinical data and scientific methods he relied on hunches and inspiration to suggest new avenues and ideas. All scientists do this to some extent. But as he turned away from bacteriology and its complicated techniques and began to work with plants his intuition became more and more dominant. In 1928 a spon-taneous visit to Wales led to the discovery of the first of the flower essences, when he brought back with him specimens of two new plants – *Impatiens glandulifera* and *Mimulus guttatus* – and prepared and tested them as he had prepared and tested so many others before. Gut feeling played a major part in his decision two years later to leave his London career and Harley Street salary and give all his time to the new system. It felt right so he believed it *was* right, despite the doubt expressed by his medical colleagues.

This period saw a rapid growth in his intuitive sense, as Weeks tells us:

> During his latter years in London, and particularly during the few weeks he had been in Wales, Bach had become aware that all his senses were quickening, becoming more fully developed. He found he was able to feel, to see and to hear things of which he had not been conscious hitherto. [...] He would say that ... no scientific appliance could work so well or give such true response as the instruments his Creator had given man in his body – his senses and his intuition.

Bach's intuition guided him to a series of propositions about the new remedies he was looking for: that they would be made from plants that grew in profusion, that the flower only would be needed, that no poisonous or primitive plants would be included in the system. He could hold a flower in his hand or on his tongue and feel its effects in his body. He literally became his own laboratory, and was able to test plants out on himself before moving on to try their effects on patients.

Later on Bach's intuition allowed him to see glimpses of things happening far away or things that were only on the point of happening. On one occasion he warned his fishermen friends in Cromer that there would be a gale in three weeks' time. Those who listened to him were careful to pull their boats and nets away from the sea to safety, and when the storm duly struck on the day Bach had named their more sceptical friends had good cause for regret. Another time he got up suddenly during a meal and went directly to where an unemployed man was about to commit suicide by jumping into the sea. He told the man that he would find work soon and sure enough the very next day the man did indeed get another job. There are many similar instances recorded in Bach's biography.

the uses of adversity

Having a purpose in life helps us to see unhappiness, pain and disappointment as challenges rather than failures. Sometimes the pain leads to insight and growth that we could not have achieved any other way. This was certainly true in the last years of Bach's life. A series of health problems led to a dramatic blossoming of his flower remedy work, one that would double the number of essences and complete the system in the space of a few short months.

Bach was living in the house at Mount Vernon by now, happy to spend the summer and winter of 1934 arranging the garden to his liking and making furniture for the empty rooms. But there were more remedies to find, and this fact announced itself to him in an entirely unexpected way when in March 1935 he was struck down with terrible sinus pains. They were so bad he felt as if he were going mad, as if he were losing his reason and might be driven to do something desperate to make the pain stop. After several days of this he was drawn to the fresh white blossoms on a cherry plum tree. The early spring sun didn't give enough heat for him to use his usual preparation method so he tried boiling up the flowering twigs instead. The tincture he produced gave him immediate relief from his loss of control, and as this went so did the physical pain.

This pattern repeated itself for all the remaining essences that he identified during the course of that spring and summer. Before each discovery he suffered the mental state for which a remedy was required, and as with the Cherry Plum state severe and painful physical symptoms often accompanied the mental condition. He endured burning rashes, hair loss, loss of vision, ulcers and even a severe haemorrhage. After he found the last remedy in August he was exhausted.

By this time people had begun to hear about the unconventional doctor in Sotwell. New patients came to see him, as well as people he had treated in the past. He also made time to teach others how to use the remedies, for he was clear that the system belonged to everyone and that all who wanted to could learn to use it. He was already working with a small team of local people who he had trained. In addition he taught visitors from outside the UK who were able to take their new knowledge back to their own countries when they left.

Perhaps somebody informed the General Medical Council of Bach's activities because he now received a letter from them. A few years before they had taken him to task for publishing an advertisement in the press in order to tell people about the essences. Now they wrote to draw to his attention the rules against working with lay assistants. He wrote back in January 1936: 'Having received the notification of the Council concerning working with unqualified assistants, it is only honourable to inform you that I am working with several, and shall continue to do so.' He expected to be struck off by return of post but the Council never replied.

Bach's last few months on earth were spent spreading news about his discoveries. He drew up a new edition of *The Twelve Healers* to include all the new essences. He also planned a lecture tour, and gave its inaugural talk in nearby Wallingford on 24 September 1936 – his fiftieth birthday. His team of assistants went on to talk in towns and villages nearby, but by the end of October Bach himself was seriously ill. On 27 November he died in his sleep.

Death is often presented in the West as 'the great leveller', the one fact that cuts us all back to size and reduces us to the dust from whence we came. But when Bach died he had finished the work that he dreamed of when he was a boy and had found a system of healing unrivalled in its simplicity, power and positivity. No death at the end of a purposeful life is ever just 'levelling'. Bach lived just as long as he had to, and walked every step of the path that led him, in the end, to where he wanted to be.

two kinds of simplicity

In his book *Simplicity*, Edward de Bono reminds us of the two things we might mean when we say that a system is simple.

❀ *First*, we might mean that it has only a few parts and that it is easy to see how it fits together. We can call this type of simplicity *simplicity-in-itself*.

❀ *Second*, we might mean that it is simple to use, so that the user can achieve complex ends with the minimum of training. We can call this kind of simplicity *ease-of-use*.

The two types of simplicity often sit at opposite ends of a seesaw. In other words simplicity-in-itself is gained at the expense of ease-of-use, and vice versa. It is easier to use a calculator to work out a square root than it is to use a slide rule, but of the two the slide rule has the simpler organisation. We can make a sledge out of a tea tray and it will be simple-in-itself, but it will be harder to steer and stop than a more complex shop-bought toboggan. We might ask an engineer to add front runners and a complicated braking system to it and so increase its ease-of-use. But as a result we will need to take it back to the engineer every time it goes wrong instead of hammering out the dents ourselves. The overall complexity involved in the home-made sledge hasn't melted away. Instead we have shifted it from one end of the seesaw (it was simple-in-itself but complex-in-use) to the other (it is complex-in-itself but easy-to-use).

The ideal sledge is fast and stable downhill, portable, easy to steer and has few moving parts. In other words it is effective while combining both types of simplicity. Things and ideas that achieve this kind of perfect balance stay around for a long time because innovations tend to make them more complex in one or both directions without adding to their effectiveness. We could add a satellite guidance system and drinks dispenser to the sledge but that doesn't make it a better sledge, i.e. better at going downhill, easier to steer, easier to understand.

Away from the world of winter sports a book is a good example of just such a balanced system. A book is made of ink, paper and glue. It is so simple-in-itself that pre-school children can happily make and illustrate their own (as long as somebody helps with the scissors). A book is also easy-to-use: just open it and read. You can put a book in your handbag, briefcase, pocket or backpack. You can read on trains, planes and boats, in parks and in hammocks, walking along, sitting down, or while eating your breakfast. You can mark your place with your shopping list or bus ticket or just fold the corner over. Books are so effective and so simple that the Internet age, which was supposed to herald the death of print, has seen more people buying and reading books than ever before. Many of the most successful commercial sites on the world-wide web are bookshops. E-books – electronic books that you read on a hand-held computer – have their place, but that place is a tiny niche compared with the vast and extending plains of the traditional reader. There will always be books, just as there will always be hammers, axes and pencils.

As we have seen, Bach talked of his thirty-eight essences as a complete system. Because there are only thirty-eight remedies it can easily be learned, understood and applied. Like the book, his system achieves the highest possible effectiveness while balancing simplicity-in-itself (the only working parts are thirty-eight simple preparations and basic self-awareness) and ease-of-use (it's easy to pick, mix and take the ones we need). This balanced simplicity is one of the system's main advantages and explains why most people still use the essences just as Bach and his lay assistants did.

adding wrinkles

It takes confidence to accept simple things at face value. If we don't have that confidence simplicity can unsettle us and lead to doubt. Perhaps we are being shallow. Perhaps we need to look further. It can't be that simple, we say, and almost before we realise it we start to add wrinkles so that once-simple techniques blossom into baroque and forbidding specialities.

Over the years a number of people have tried the effect of adding metaphorical satellite systems and drink dispensers to Bach's work. One German therapist divides the body up into sections, each related to different essences, so that somebody wanting to use the essences needs his map of the body to apply the right flower. Another introduces sets of so-called 'new combinations', such as Clematis-plus-Scleranthus and Clematis-plus-Star of Bethlehem. His descriptions of these mix up the indications for each single flower, so they are completely pointless, but they do add a lot of complexity. Instead of looking through thirty-eight remedies for those that apply to our situation we have to ferret through hundreds of pages in search of a combination that seems a reasonable match. (While we do so we might wonder why his few thousand combinations should be more valid than the hundreds of millions that he *doesn't* mention...) Other therapists decorate the system with chakras (you have to learn the chakras before you select remedies) or astrology (you have to draw a birth chart before you select remedies) or homoeopathy (you have to be a homoeopath to use remedies). The result every time is the same. There is less simplicity-in-itself and less ease-of-use, and no compensating increase in effectiveness.

All this is nothing compared with the muddle over dosage instructions. Mystique and personal prejudice have obfuscated something that should be so simple it hardly needs thinking about. Three drops three times a day, seven drops morning and night, nine drops in the morning and seven three times a day, four drops before and after meals, two drops undiluted for three days followed by two weeks diluted at eight drops a day... No wonder many people feel like Alison Hudd, whose osteopath used dowsing to create a customised dosage pattern. 'She gave me very complicated instructions as to how many drops and at what time of day to take them. I found it quite stressful remembering her instructions and organising my day around them.'

Taking essences shouldn't be stressful or complicated. We might agree once more with de Bono, who lists a number of reasons why people can be attracted to unnecessary complexity. These include snob value (espousing a complicated idea makes us seem culturally and intellectually superior) and self-interest (complication creates a job for the initiated expert). A kinder view is that these theorists lack the confidence they need to accept simplicity and grow with it. We could no doubt suggest remedies to help.

When we compare Bach's early and late writings on the remedies we can see how his idea of development went the other way. He tended to start with complex ideas drawn from many different traditions, and slowly got simpler and more focused as his confidence in his findings grew. We can trace this change in many ways, but I have chosen to concentrate on two areas: the relationship of the remedies to physical disease, and their relationship to astrology.

physical symptoms

Bach's main mention of physical symptoms in connection with emotional states comes in *Heal Thyself*, where he writes: 'any type of illness from which we may suffer will guide us to the discovery of the fault which lies behind our affliction. ... the very part of the body affected is no accident, but is in accordance with the law of cause and effect, and again will be a guide to help us.'

Unhistorical reading of this statement has led to a lot of mis-understanding. The commonest is the forging of spurious relation-ships between 'stiff' remedies like Beech, Rock Water and Water Violet and the stiffness of stiff necks, frozen shoulders, paralysis and arthritis.

Bach was a doctor, trained to look for physical symptoms as an aid to diagnosis. In his orthodox research into vaccines and even later when he turned towards homoeopathy he was preoccupied wholly or in part with physical illness. He wrote *Heal Thyself* in June and July 1930. He had just three essences to work with and had only recently discovered the sun method of preparation (see chapter 5, page 126). The dust of his London laboratory still clung to his shoes. With his long training in physical illness it was natural for him to assume that physical symptoms would continue to be relevant to his new work, if in an attenuated and symbolic form.

This soon changed. As he added more essences to the system Bach realised that the connection he had assumed between particular flowers and particular illnesses simply wasn't there. Within a few months of completing *Heal Thyself* he wrote an article on the new essences he had discovered that summer, in which he was firmly against diagnosis by means of physical symptoms. 'It matters not what may be the physical disease of our patient,' he wrote, 'we have to com-prehend to which of the above types he belongs.' The new system bypassed the physical and could and should be selected only on the basis of how people felt. Selecting using physical symptoms was more complex and plain didn't work. The person with arthritis who insist-ed on telling all her neighbours about it needed Heather, not Rock Water; the person with stiff shoulders might not need Beech at all, but Mimulus to help him ask his boss for a new office chair, or Vervain to help him turn off and relax, or Oak or Elm for being overworked. Towards the end Bach said that his lay helpers were better at selecting remedies than he was because they didn't have to try to forget years of medical training. They found it easier than he did to ignore the physical symptoms of the people they saw. In this sense their use of his system was actually purer and more effective than his own.

astrology

At one stage Bach believed there might be a similar direct relationship between astrology and flower essences. We know this from a couple of scattered references. In an essay published in the *Homoeopathic World* in February 1930 he mentions 'the planetary influences' as one of the factors that may have to be considered in order to produce the most potent essences possible. And in a letter he wrote to some friends in 1933 he says the flower remedy system looked like it would 'assist vastly in the purification and understanding of astrology'. In the same letter, however, he is careful not to go too far: 'I am being very cautious as regards astrology, and that is why one left out the signs and the months in the first *Twelve Healers*. … I do not wish to be associated with anything dogmatic, until one is sure.'

Astrology and the remedies are both based on the assumption that we can classify all human beings by combining a limited number of criteria: planets and constellations in one system, remedies in another. With twelve remedies in his first series and twelve signs of the zodiac Bach must have felt the coincidence was worthy of investigation. Indeed, he held on to the thought that the first twelve remedies were 'special' even when he had discovered more than twelve. *The Twelve Healers and Four Helpers* and *The Twelve Healers and Seven Helpers*, published in 1933 and 1934 respectively, both treat the 'helper' remedies as adjuncts to the 'healers', reserved for people whose illnesses have gone on for some time and who have not improved after taking the correct remedy from the original twelve.

Bach abandoned this structure when he prepared the final edition of his book, *The Twelve Healers and Other Remedies*. There are clearly more than twelve type or personality essences (think of Vine,

Beech, Oak, Heather, none of which was in the original twelve), and the only reason that he kept the title 'Twelve Healers' was that he knew his readers were familiar with it. We can tell the original twelve from the other twenty-six because an asterisk marks them out, but nowhere are they given any priority over the other remedies. Even the asterisk was added by the publisher, not by Bach.

What happened to astrology and its purification?

I don't want to defend or attack the validity of astrology (or any other belief system) in this book. Astrologers have fought their corner for thousands of years and need no help from the likes of me. But whether we believe or disbelieve in astrology I hope we can all agree that in part it is a way of using categories to describe people. Astrologers use a language (signs of the zodiac and planet position) to describe somebody's emotional and spiritual state. 'John is a Virgo' is supposed to tell us something about John. Remedy users do the same, using a language made up of flower essences: 'John is a bit of a Vine with overtones of Wild Rose' *says* something. We can describe the same person using both languages, but that doesn't mean the two languages contain exactly the same words.

It might be clearer what I mean if we look at a more familiar kind of language, spoken language. If I want to describe my wrecked car I can use French and say '*elle est dans les choux*' or I can use English and say 'it's up the spout'. The two phrases mean the same thing, but they contain elements that have nothing to do with each other. I can't translate the French description into English by concentrating on the words '*dans*' and '*choux*' because the result in English – 'it's in the cabbages' – paints an entirely false picture of my car's current state. Instead I need to look at the car, see that it is wrecked, and express this in whichever language I am using. For the same reason, if I want to describe John using astrology and flower remedies the place I need to start is always John. And the two descriptions I end up with, both accurate in their own ways, will contain different elements with no direct correspondence between them.

For this reason we need to be very cautious (as Bach was) about drawing simple and direct analogies between any one flower (Scleranthus, say) and any one star sign (Libra). Like different languages, the systems don't fit together in the same way, and the terms 'Libra' and 'Scleranthus' perform different functions despite their apparent similarities. Pretending otherwise does a disservice to both traditions. Clearly Bach saw things this way as well. The signs of the zodiac never did appear in any edition of *The Twelve Healers*. The system is complete, and with no mention of astrology.

scaffolding

Bach published his findings at every stage so that people might benefit from them at once, even though he knew that he might have to revise them in a few months. To try to prevent confusion he always told his publishers to destroy remaining stocks of *The Twelve Healers* as each new edition came to press. On one occasion he even had a bonfire in the garden at Mount Vernon, much to the horror of his friends, and burnt most of his notebooks, letters and personal papers. For in Bach's eyes these notes and ideas and theories could only cause confusion. He saw them as scaffolding, necessary to help construct the building but no longer needed – a positive hindrance even – once the house was complete and ready for living in. In place of all the theory the final version of *The Twelve Healers* was a model of practical simplicity.

This movement from complex ideas to a final simple statement flies in the face of the general rule, which is for systems to become more complex as exceptions and special cases are taken into account. Bach's commitment to simplicity was extraordinary. He distilled his work into its most fundamental form. He stripped away every trace of unnecessary decoration and speculation. It's as if he were some kind of Picasso-in-reverse, starting with the huge canvas of *La Guernica* and deconstructing it back to the first pen and ink sketch, the simplest and purest expression of his vision.

His focus on the ideal and most practical form of his work rather than on what most of us think of as 'posterity' – the number of works, the weight on the shelves – helped Bach create something unique, a perfect tool that has proved not to need revision. Its simplicity makes the system easier to learn and easier to use and easier to introduce to other people. We only need to know the essences and have a basic understanding of the way we feel. Healing is available to you and your doctor and your priest and your grocer and your tarot reader – to everybody, regardless of their beliefs and prejudices. But let us come back to what Bach said: 'they who will obtain the greatest benefit from this God-sent Gift will be those who keep it pure as it is; free from science, free from theories, for everything in Nature is simple.' This says more, that using the system in its pure and simple form will actually have better results *for the user*. Why is this?

iv ❀ living today

Seize the day, never trust the next.

– Horace, Roman poet, 65–8 BC

seven remedies to seize the day

Now comes only once. If we miss it we will never live it. Yet this simple lesson is one of the hardest we have to learn. So much of our thinking is else-where – stuck in the past, fixed on the future, worrying over things that may never happen, sunk into indifference or lack of attention – that we miss an infinity of nows every day. The things we might have done and the heights we might have reached run away from us like water through open hands. To slow down time we need to focus on the present and feel a sense of commit-ment to every second of our lives. We need to think of each moment as a wonderful meal and savour every mouthful, whether bitter or sweet.

Edward Bach's group of essences against insufficient interest in the present helps us focus on the now that comes once. It includes seven essences.

- ❀ **White Chestnut** helps to calm our minds when they run in circles around niggling worries. It helps us put aside intrusive thoughts and engage more fully in what we are doing.
- ❀ **Wild Rose** is the flower of zest and enthusiasm. It helps when we start to drift and feel that life is passing us by.
- ❀ **Honeysuckle** brings us away from the past and into the present. It helps when we get caught up in past regrets or past pleasures to such an extent that we no longer expect to find joy in the present.

✿ **Olive** helps restore strength when we are so tired that we lose the ability to show interest.

✿ **Chestnut Bud** is to do with experience and learning. In the negative state we repeat mistakes because we have not noticed or taken responsibility for our actions.

✿ **Clematis** is for when our thoughts stray into the future. Lost in our dreams we fail to act and so lose the chance to make our dreams come true. Clematis roots us in reality.

✿ **Mustard** is for when we lose consciousness of the joy we have in life. We feel an unaccountable depression – nothing has gone wrong but we still feel down – and the flower helps us rise out of this and feel how blessed we are.

'They must often change who would be constant in happiness or wisdom,' said the Chinese philosopher Confucius; but change is valueless unless we can notice and learn from it. Being preoccupied to the extent that we don't notice our growth is the same as being half asleep. The remedies in this group are a wake-up call.

> I have become more sensitive since taking the Bach remedies, even in my reaction to atmospheric variations and weather changes. This is due to encouraging and developing greater general awareness. Things that I didn't take too much notice of I now register more consciously. – Miki Hayashi

calm your thoughts: white chestnut

'I did my work,' said the sleepless man with a querulous intonation.

'And this is the price?'

'Yes.'

For a little while the two remained without speaking.

'You cannot imagine the craving for rest that I feel – a hunger and thirst. For six long days, since my work was done, my mind has been a whirlpool, swift, unprogressive and incessant, a torrent of thoughts leading nowhere, spinning round swift and steady ... Spin, spin, spin, spin. It goes round and round, round and round for ever more.'

H.G. Wells, *When the Sleeper Wakes*

There are echoes of stillness in the horse chestnut tree *Aesculus hippocastanum*, from which the White Chestnut remedy comes. One is in the flowering candles, which stand erect and motionless on a thick central stem. Another is in the fruit of the tree, whose spiky, busy shell breaks open to show a round smooth shiny conker inside – an image if we choose to see it of stillness beneath a troubled surface. The stillness is always there. To find it we have to open up and let go of our worries. We have to stay quiet and not jump to conclusions. Meditation, chanting and ritual all aim to move the mind closer to the stillness and wisdom within; Bach was only one of many teachers who have spoken of the need above all to *quiet the mind*.

In a negative White Chestnut this is precisely what we struggle to do. Practitioners often describe White Chestnut thoughts as worrying, which is accurate but sometimes misleading because we tend to equate worry with anxiety. Real White Chestnut worrying has more to do with what dogs do to bones and to sheep. It means keeping on, not giving up, continually coming back to the same thing. As with most mental activity this is not always and necessarily bad in itself. The mind's ability to worry over a problem gives it a way of testing possible solutions. But in a White Chestnut state we lose control of our worrying so that it becomes an end in itself. Our thoughts run away with us and wear themselves into a groove. One thought leads to another and back to the first with no resolution or way out. Sometimes the groove replays past events and we think back over things that happened during the day, or go over and over what we said, what she said and what we should have said. Other times our thoughts build around the future so that it is tomorrow's ifs, ands and buts that circle in our head. Or it could be something unreal or unconnected to our own life that sets the wheel spinning, such as something said on television or a remark overheard in the street.

Practitioners associate the White Chestnut state with insomnia because a worrying mind is not quiet enough to allow sleep to come. The connection isn't exclusive, however, and insomnia can have other causes. Even where active thoughts are definitely the cause this could indicate Agrimony (repressed thoughts returning in the quiet moments) or Vervain (unable to switch off and planning tomorrow's activities). When in doubt the telltale sign is the quality of circularity: if the thoughts go round and round without getting us anywhere then White Chestnut is the right flower.

White Chestnut worry is at its most destructive when we are already out of balance in another area. Any pre-existing negative emotions intensify if we worry over them and find no solutions. If we are depressed, for example, we may pick one particular aspect of depression to worry over. It may be tiredness, so that a Hornbeam state develops into a new main problem. Or it may be our appearance, leading to a Crab Apple mood. Instead of isolating tiredness as a factor in depression and then doing something about it – taking exercise or eating better, for example – the White Chestnut state makes us feel helpless so that we sink further into the state we have identified. It is because worry so often accompanies and exacerbates other negative states that White Chestnut is one of the most frequently used of helper remedies, and may kick off a process of healing that involves moving back through underlying layers of negativity.

I was getting a lot of unwanted and worrying thoughts and was unable to sleep at night. A mental chatter would keep on and on, never resting, the same problem would just churn around in my mind. The remedy that really helped me was White Chestnut.
– Claire Hingley

One of the most impressive effects I have experienced was when I took White Chestnut one evening during a course. I knew the day's work would be going around in my head and stop me from getting to sleep. I lay in my bed for about twenty minutes, thoughts whizzing around with no sign of abating, but then it was as though someone reached into my head and pulled out all my thoughts. It was wonderful and I slept like a log. – Lynn Hinton

a london street

I was about nine years old. It was summer and I was home from school so it must have been a late afternoon in June or July. I walked down the concrete steps in front of our house and turned left. I was walking next to my mother. We were going to a shop on the other side of the block where we lived and I was looking forward to digging around in the cheap plastic toys while my mother bought whatever she wanted to buy.

Flying ants covered the whole of the baked pavement on our side of the street. They settled on my shoes and trousers, taking short random flights into the air. It was impossible not to tread on some of them. The street smelled of heat and dust, the sun beat down on my head and a million tiny lives flew and settled all around.

The intensity of that day has never left me. In my head the yellow light is like a Van Gogh sunflower. I can smell the melting tar in the street and taste the sweat on my lips and the back of my hand. The teeming of life hits me like a hammer. Nothing particular was happening – I was drifting along with my mother to a local shop, just for something to do – but I saw and felt every moment with the clear-sightedness and the full five senses of childhood. When other more dramatic events are forgotten in old age I will still taste the dust of that long-ago London afternoon in the 1960s and smell the paving stones and hear the flick of wings in the air.

feel alive: wild rose

There is a world of difference between how I felt in that 1960s summer – drifting yet completely alive, curious and open and recording – and what happens when we drift but forget awareness. And this difference measures the gap between the positive and negative Wild Rose states.

In a negative Wild Rose state we feel that life is passing us by. We drift from moment to moment and place to place and find no joy in anything. We are committed to nothing. We lack motivation and willpower and because of this find it difficult to change. We are not deeply depressed about our situation, for we may feel so disconnected that the power of strong negative emotions has left us. Instead we suffer a chronic, low-lying feeling of apathy. We resign ourselves to the monotony of life and to putting up with the things that happen to us. We surrender to illness and pain and pleasure with the same lack of enthusiasm. We may resist change, though never in a very active way. Our gesture is a shrug of the shoulders: 'Oh well, what can I do? I'll just have to accept it.'

Taking Wild Rose helps fuel a sense of purpose and a desire to grow. It removes apathy and teaches instead the art of purposeful drifting. In the positive Wild Rose state we pay full attention to our lives moment by moment and drink juice from every second. We don't have to try. We relax and the world comes to us. We are lilies of the field, neither toiling nor spinning, yet still arrayed in and conscious of glory. We are children, learning all the time, brimming with curiosity, wonder and delight, our open faces shouting a joyous 'yes' to life.

> I can remember vividly, as a child, finding some beautiful pale pink roses growing in the hedge in the lane. I was desperate to pick them to take home to keep, but was disappointed to find that as soon as I picked them the petals fell. As soon as the flower was cut off from its life source it gave up, having no energy or desire to survive. I can remember feeling so sad that this little rose had withered and died but, worse still, I was the cause. How lovely it has been to find that Dr Bach had already discovered such healing powers in these little roses. My guilt has eased. – Jill Head

a memory nightmare

In Russia chance blessed a newspaper reporter called Shereshevskii with a remarkable memory. He could memorise a list of seventy words in minutes and recall it perfectly fifteen years later, forwards or backwards, along with details like the place where he first heard the list, who was present, where they sat and what they wore. He could recall sensations too, with great precision and in all their glory, as if they were present now. He could lower or raise his pulse dramatically just by thinking about going to sleep or running for a train, or simultaneously raise the temperature of one hand and lower that of the other by imagining one over a stove and the other holding ice.

For years the subject of research by psychologists, Shereshevskii's gift ended up as a curse. He was unable to forget. In his later life he had accumulated so many memories that everything around him evoked images, tastes, voices and smells from the past. He couldn't work or read or talk or think in the present because of the press of recall. He couldn't even draw lessons from his past or see the pattern of his life. He recalled all the single incidents so perfectly and in such detail that they were unavailable to generalisation.

Shereshevskii the man drowned in his memories.

accept your past: honeysuckle

The lingering perfume of the flowers and the plant's association with cottage gardens forge a natural link between the Honeysuckle remedy and nostalgia. If only things could be as they once were, we think. I will never know joy like that again. This is one version of the Honeysuckle state. Another is when we are consumed by regrets: That is where it all went wrong. If only I could go back to do things differently. Nostalgic or regretful, having our thoughts anchored in the past drags our minds away from the present and the future. Consequently we will not plan or try to improve things. Ours is a sad state of being lost in memories, a more everyday version of Shereshevskii's nightmare inability to forget.

Often we associate the Honeysuckle state with old people. There is some truth in this. Popular culture builds around youth and physical energy and tends to marginalise people once they are no longer young. Memories grow more attractive as present opportunities shrink. And at the same time, whether for cultural or biological reasons, memories of childhood and young adulthood return more vividly as the years go by. But the Honeysuckle state does not spare children either. The homesickness of a child sent away to a new school is also a typical Honeysuckle emotion.

The common name 'honeysuckle' is based on the assumption that bees suck honey from the sweet-smelling flowers of *Lonicera caprifolium*. This is wrong. Bees get nothing from the honeysuckle, just as we get nothing from our negative Honeysuckle memories. The other common name for the plant, woodbine, comes from its habit of winding itself around trees. Woodbine can strangle trees and stop them from growing; again there is an obvious analogy to the effect of Honeysuckle memories on the people who are gripped by them. By extension we can say that the Honeysuckle remedy is about drawing the honey from our past without getting bound up in it. In the positive state we can generalise our experiences into rules and principles. We can move on from old griefs and regrets, see them in today's perspective rather than yesterday's, and not allow their shadow to darken today. We can find goodness in past suffering and draw strength from old weaknesses. 'No thoughts of past errors must ever depress us,' said Bach. 'They are over and finished, and the knowledge thus gained will help to avoid a repetition of them.'

grow your strength: olive

In the negative Olive state we are exhausted and need to find new reserves. Olive reminds us that we can always find more energy within ourselves and puts us back in contact with that energy. It shares its characteristics with the fruit of the olive tree and the oil made from it. All in their different ways promote health and vitality.

We often think of the negative Olive state as being the result of hard physical work. But it is just as likely to come *after* the body has struggled against a disease, or *after* some mental effort such as studying, thinking or worrying over something. Emotional exhaustion is also an Olive state when it comes *after* trauma or the chronic erosion of family arguments or stress at work. The key is this word *after*: in an Olive state there has always been effort and exertion at some level to cause the tiredness. This contrasts with the Hornbeam state (see page 46) in which tiredness comes at the mere thought of making an effort – in other words, *before* we enter the struggle.

Olive alone will always help us recover in the short term. But we may need to look for other essences if our behaviour often leaves us tired. Constant or repeated exhaustion suggests that we need to develop some personal quality that will help us measure our lives better. Dogged Oaks, enthusiastic Vervains, helpful Centauries and party-going Agrimonies – all of us can drift into out-of-balance lifestyles that leave us tired and needing respite. In this state Olive is a helper remedy; the 'cure' lies with the flower that will rebalance the cause of the tiredness.

The olive tree has been known as a symbol of peace way back into ancient times. Even today if we hold out a metaphorical olive branch to somebody it is a sign that we wish to make peace. This reminds us of a second positive potential of the Olive remedy that is sometimes overlooked: its ability to bring us back to a place of rest. In an extreme Olive state we have suffered so much that we take no pleasure in daily life. Everything is impossibly hard work, even staying quiet and falling asleep. Olive allows us to withdraw into ourselves and find respite. We can let go of our suffering and trust our bodies and minds to find the strength they need without our conscious help.

When I take the Olive remedy there is no sudden burst of energy like you might expect with conventional medicine. Instead it's as though I have forgotten all about being tired. Only some time later do I realise that the fatigue has been lifted. – Stuart Guffogg

I find Olive an amazing remedy for tiredness. It seems to wake me up almost immediately and I use it frequently. – Elaine More

learning

As babies we know from birth how to get the things we need and avoid the things that could kill us. We hold on to our mothers. We suck at breast or bottle. We cry to get warmth or food or comfort. We turn away from shapes that could mean danger. We could describe these abilities as instinctive cleverness, for they do not require any thought or experience. Nobody needs to demonstrate these skills to us and we don't need to practise them. We just do them.

True intelligence is of a different order. It means adapting to our surroundings so as to function better, and adaptation in the course of a single lifetime – as opposed to Darwinian adaptation over the lifetime of a species – involves learning. We have learned when we can react differently to new situations based on our experience of what happened in the past. If we didn't develop in this way we would always turn aside and cry for help when a shape appeared. Thanks to learning we can react differently depending on whether somebody tosses a ball or a grenade to us. The more effectively we learn from our experiences and from those of the people around us the further along our own personal evolutionary path we can travel. For learning and growth, from this point of view, are the same thing.

According to the teacher and writer Guy Claxton the most effective forms of learning are often slow and largely unconscious. They involve pulling patterns from experience and developing a *feel* for how to do things, rather than sitting down and learning conscious rules. Driving lessons work on this principle. We don't learn about brakes and the clutch in a classroom. Instead we sit inside a car and after a basic introduction ('this is the steering wheel, this is the brake') we start to drive. We get more guidance from the instructor as we go – and a guarantee of safety – but we do the actual learning by registering the effects of each movement we make and gradually building up a model of what good driving *feels* like. As we become more competent we start to perform the right actions without thinking about it.

Unconscious learning is not restricted to mechanical skills like driving. It also applies to more intellectual abilities. In scientific research, for example, hunches tell scientists where to look next. Trying to discover new things using set logical routines is slow and ineffective compared with the sudden intuitive leap towards a beautiful, right-feeling hypothesis. A crucial part of scientific training is therefore the slow and unconscious development of intuition. Beyond the formulae and maths in the textbooks student scientists are learning by trial and error what good science *feels* like. Language learning provides another example. We can't learn to speak a foreign language well using textbooks and sentence rules alone. Instead the best way to learn Chinese is to live in China until we get a *feel* for how Chinese works. And as we all know, the best language learners are children, who never consult a grammar or a dictionary but just live in the culture and absorb the language like a sponge. At seven or eight years old a child will speak her native tongue with a grace and fluency that no scholar could begin to match.

A friend of mine read a lot as a child and developed a *feel* for good writing. Later as a student he enjoyed the enviable ability to sit down in an exam and create an essay without having to plan it first. But then, aged fifteen or so, he began preparing for more formal assessments. His teacher stopped lecturing on the subject and began teaching how to write essays. She laid down strict rational rules showing how to plan the introduction, the main points and the conclusion. As a good student, my friend tried to answer the questions using the teacher's rules when he sat his first mock exam. And suddenly he found he couldn't write. Everything was on crutches. His words limped across the page like wounded men. The argument tied itself in knots and reached no conclusion. And for the first time he failed.

His experience points up an interesting phenomenon with which we are all familiar: that becoming conscious of our unconsciously learned rules of thumb can actually make our performance worse. If we get into our car years after passing the test and try to drive in a conscious way, thinking of every control and action before we carry it out – 'this is the steering wheel, this is the brake' – we will not drive anything like as well. If we speak Chinese like a native but decide one day to think out every sentence before we say it we will find ourselves tongue-tied.

My friend abandoned the rules and went back to doing things that felt right, and he passed his exams. This doesn't mean that the rules the teacher provided were wrong, or that nobody needs rules. Unconscious knowledge helps us deal with repetitions of the same situation – reversing a car is always reversing a car – but if we want to drive an articulated lorry instead of a car we need to be able to apply what we know about car driving to the new situation. That way if the handbrake isn't where we expect it or the mirrors are in different places we won't be completely stumped. We will be conscious of the fact that they must be there somewhere and take the time to look for them. Knowing what to look for and being able to conceptualise processes gives us expertise at living and puts us more in control of the unexpected. And when things don't feel right we have a better chance of finding the cause of the problem. At university my friend struggled to adapt his writing style to the formal needs of a history degree. This time the rational hints in a writing manual proved useful. They helped him to see where he was going wrong and correct his technique for this new form.

As with everything, then, balance is the key. The most effective learning comes when we are good at building up unconscious patterns and equally good at drawing conscious rules from them. Unconsciously and consciously we need to pay attention so as to learn from our lives.

learn: chestnut bud

Chestnut Bud comes into play when we fail to see patterns in our lives – consciously or unconsciously – and so fail to learn from experience. We can see negative Chestnut Bud behaviour in people who repeat their mistakes: the woman who forges relationships with one violent and abusive man after another; the man who leaves a job he hates for a similar job in a similar company; the student who fails her exam for the same reason that she failed a year ago. Chestnut Bud would also help the alcoholic's daughter who uses drugs to get through her dad's funeral, and the gambling sons of the man ruined by his incautious approach to business. They too could avoid their mistakes if they could find patterns in the experiences of other people. I remember seeing both types of Chestnut Bud people on a hospital cancer ward. The waiting area by the lifts was always taken up by smokers, some of them visitors and some of them patients in their dressing gowns, frail and barely able to breathe, but still cadging matches and lighting up 'to relax'.

All wisdom is based on experience and the uses we make of it. Taking Chestnut Bud opens us up to growth. We don't forget things as soon as they happen. We hold events in our minds long enough to evaluate and learn from them. We see the link between our thoughts, decisions and actions and the consequences that arise from them. We learn based on past experience what *feels* right and can act rightly based on that knowledge. This gives us a firm basis on which to plan our futures and move forward.

The Chestnut Bud and White Chestnut essences both come from the same tree. The buds make the first remedy and the fully opened flowers the second. When making the Chestnut Bud essence we need to use the right kind of tree – 'make certain the trees are the white chestnut and not the red chestnut,' writes Nora Weeks – but unfortunately we are working blind because we can't see the colour of the flowers yet. Perhaps Weeks learned the hard way and was keen to pass her experiences on to beginners.

build your dreams: clematis

'You only offer me cold materialism, life on the earth with all its hardships and sorrows, and there far away is my dream, my ideal. Do you blame me if I follow it?'

And Clematis came along and said, 'Are your ideals God's ideals? Are you sure that you are serving Him Who made you, Who created you, Who gave you your life, or are you listening just to some other human being who is trying to claim you, and so you are forgetting that you are a son of God with all His Divinity within your soul, and instead of this glorious reality you are being lured away by just some other human being?

'I know how we long to fly away to more wonderful realms, but, brothers of the human world, let us first fulfil our duty and even not our duty but our joy, and may you adorn the places where you live and strive to make them beautiful as I endeavour to make the hedges glorious, so that they have called me the travellers' joy.'

Edward Bach

We need to have dreams and ambitions and look forward to future happiness because that helps us feel alive and positive about tomorrow. But once again it's a question of balance. Dreams only help if they cast light on today. Dreaming by itself will never build a future. This is the lesson that Clematis has for us.

My first job was as a clerk in the civil service. I hated everything about it: the files, the desk, the telephone, the telex, the meaninglessness of buying belt buckles for Brunei and military medals for Mombasa. To escape I took long lunch-breaks in a dusty park by the Thames next to the Houses of Parliament in Westminster. There I would wander around talking to myself, giving imaginary interviews to journalists explaining how I had managed to break away from my humdrum life and become a famous rock star. After an hour or an hour and a half of monologue I went back to prison and an afternoon of clock-watching. That was negative Clematis – fantasy, imagination and no attempt to change things.

In a negative Clematis state we use our dreams as a way of escaping from our current circumstances. If something happens that we don't want to deal with we avoid it. We break off and fly away from ourselves at the barest touch of wind, just like the feathery seeds of *Clematis vitalba*. Our escape is a fantasy that leaves our actual situation unchanged. Daydreaming turns to vacancy and lack of will, so much so that Bach characterised the negative Clematis state as 'a polite form of suicide'. The true Clematis type stands wide-eyed and doesn't hear what people say to her. Her thoughts are miles away, up in the clouds and away with the fairies. She breaks off in the middle of what she is saying and loses the thread. She may feel drowsy or lose consciousness or fall asleep easily or sleep a great deal – all signs of a mind not focused on the present.

The positive is seen in those creative people who build on their ability to dream vividly, to fantasise and allow the mind to play in all the fields of possibility and impossibility. In the positive state we know that the way forward is to make use of today. We take practical steps to make our dreams come true. We don't just dream of being a great artist, we grip our brush and put paint on the canvas. If our ambition is to help animals we take biology options at school and talk to a bank manager about financing our way through veterinary college. If we want our children to have successful careers and be happy and balanced people we get involved in their lives now, reading to them and helping them to grow. Positive Clematis is a practical dreamer, her gaze fixed on the stars and the life to come but her feet on the ground and moving. Her dreams take root in real life and for that very reason there is no limit to what she can achieve.

Throughout my lonely childhood I lived inside my imagination. My daydreaming continued into adulthood as a form of escape. I wasn't truly living. Clematis helped me to break this long-held pattern. I turned the creativity outward into the writing of poetry and had a substantial amount of work published. – Susan

Five years ago I moved and had to leave some things in storage as the place I was moving to was rented and full of the landlord's furniture. I kept saying that the place I was living was only temporary. When I *next* moved I would get my things back and have this and that in such a way and so on. I said this to myself for five years, until Clematis came along. Now the landlord has been around to take his furniture away and I have mine out of storage and my own curtains hanging in the windows. I am so much happier. Previously I hated being here as I was living in an imaginary house elsewhere. I am now planning future things instead of living in a dream world. – Louise

I was the daydreamer at school and even now I miss out on a lot
of conversation and TV when I drift off to other things. I need to
make a conscious effort to bring my mind to the here and now.
I also have the habit of needing regular sleep and always drop
into a deep sleep on the train home from work. – J.C.

It didn't take too long to realise that I am a Clematis type, and
I took the remedy last June for about three weeks. My ability to
concentrate and take things in is greatly enhanced, to a degree
I would have given anything for when a student – I was always
dreaming in lectures and had a short attention span. Also there
is the very hard-to-explain feeling of being *together* as a person.
– David Brandon

find joy in life: mustard

In sooth, I know not why I am so sad:
It wearies me; you say it wearies you;
But how I caught it, found it, or came by it,
What stuff 'tis made of, whereof it is born,
I am to learn;
And such a want-wit sadness makes of me,
That I have much ado to know myself.

> – William Shakespeare, *The Merchant of Venice*, Act 1, Scene 1

The path is a bedrock of inner joy and serenity. We can feel it under the soles
of our feet as long as we remain on track. When something bad happens and
blows us off the path and into the swamp of despondency there are various
essences that can help to get us back on course and back to firm ground. And
when there seems to be no reason, when everything in our lives is going well
but we still lose touch with our joy, when like Shakespeare's Antonio we know
not why we are sad, then we can consider Mustard.

Practitioners often describe the negative Mustard state as if it were a natural and inevitable phenomenon – a black cloud, a thick fog, or the fall of night – even the word 'depression' sounds as if it has been borrowed from the weather forecast. This reflects the helplessness we feel when we get down for no reason. Melancholy seems to come and go in its own good time, like the rain, and all we can do is sit through it and hope it won't last long. We retire into ourselves and our thoughts grow inwards and away from the light.

The Mustard flower is a sun dance, something we can do to dispel the thunderclouds and make the light come out sooner. It gives us a feel for the joy in our lives. It helps us remember the big eternal positives – life and its intrinsic values – as well as the small pleasures that come and go, so we can live in and for both in the same way a happy child does. Mustard reawakens our interest in life. Peace comes over us and we can resist gloom and depression because at heart we *know* we are well and that we are born to be happy and whole.

I felt that one day there would be a way out of the black hole, but at that time did not know what it would be. When I first read about Mustard it was reassuring to know that what I was experiencing was already a recognised feeling and that a very simple natural remedy was available to help me. – Lynn Hall

I suffered regularly from black depressions for seventeen years. I am happy to say that Mustard knocked that on the head! At least, once I had the sense to take it continuously for a few months rather than just when I was actually suffering. – Alice Walkingshaw

5 ❦ peaks and paradigms

peak experiences

In 1964, a few years after *Towards a Psychology of Being*, Abraham Maslow talked more about transcendence in another book. *Religions, Values, and Peak Experiences* compared the mystical visions experienced by prophets and the founders of religion with similar states reported by artists and ordinary men and women. Maslow called these states *peak experiences*, and found they tended to be the same regardless of creed or belief. They were flashes of insight, overwhelming feelings of meaning, unity and completeness that gave the sense of purpose and belonging that self-actualising people sought. Maslow hypothesised that peak experiences were natural psychological events common to all human beings, although different cultures have interpreted them in different ways.

Perhaps the easiest way to explain a peak experience is to give some examples. Literature is full of them. In *La nausée*, John-Paul Sartre's narrator goes through a peak experience while he is wandering aimlessly at dusk. A man filled with disgust and a distaste for existence, he happens to see the light of the Callebotte lighthouse come on – it is the first light to come on in the darkened town – and hears a child exclaim at the sight. Suddenly, inexplicably, life has meaning. It is as if the electrical illumination and the child's cry of wonder find an echo in his spirit, so that a sense of wonder and enlightenment grows within him almost despite himself. 'I am happy,' he writes, and there is a strange confusion in the realisation that nothing at all, the simple turning of a light switch, can bring unity and contentment into his discontented life. Hermann Hesse's narrator in *Steppenwolf* goes through a similar experience in a café. In his case the trigger is music, which transports him from his humdrum surroundings to a point where he flies through heaven and sees God. 'I dropped all my defences and was afraid of nothing,' he writes. 'I accepted all things and to all things I gave up my heart.'

The suddenness of these experiences is typical, as is the sense of acceptance and universal love. And often, as in *Steppenwolf* and *La nausée*, the peak experience is in stark contrast to a more fragmented and evil view of life.

Here is a third example, from Samuel Taylor Coleridge's *Ancient Mariner*. The albatross he shot hangs from his neck. He stands on deck surrounded by dead men, feeling disgust at his own life and at the life in the sea around him:

> The many men, so beautiful!
> And they all dead did lie:
> And a thousand thousand slimy things
> Lived on; and so did I.
>
> I looked upon the rotting sea,
> And drew my eyes away;
> I looked upon the rotting deck,
> And there the dead men lay.
>
> I looked to heaven and tried to pray;
> But or ever a prayer had gusht,
> A wicked whisper came, and made
> My heart as dry as dust.

The wicked whisper, the mariner's inability to connect with his own or other forms of life, stops him from praying. But a few verses further on he too achieves the sudden insight that accepts everything. And in accepting everything he moves back towards a state of grace:

Beyond the shadow of the ship,
I watched the water-snakes:
They moved in tracks of shining white,
And when they reared, the elfish light
Fell off in hoary flakes.

Within the shadow of the ship
I watched their rich attire:
Blue, glossy green, and velvet black,
They coiled and swam; and every track
Was a flash of golden fire.

O happy living things! no tongue
Their beauty might declare:
A spring of love gushed from my heart
And I blessed them unaware:
Sure my kind saint took pity on me,
And I blessed them unaware.

The self-same moment I could pray;
And from my neck so free
The Albatross fell off, and sank
Like lead into the sea.

Lest we think that peak experiences only happen in fiction and poetry we turn now to some personal accounts. In *Reason for Hope* the scientist and environmental campaigner Jane Goodall describes two such moments. The first was in Paris in 1974, in the cathedral of Notre-Dame. A wedding party occupied one remote corner of the vast building. Otherwise there were few people around. She was gazing up at the Rose Window when the organ struck up J.S. Bach's *Toccata and Fugue in D minor*. The combination of the place, the stillness, then the dance of music lifted her up. It was, in her words, 'a suddenly captured moment of eternity' during which the essential rightness of the universe became apparent.

The second happened in 1981. Goodall had been caught in the heart of a tropical thunderstorm and had taken refuge under a palm frond. Above her the family of chimpanzees she was following sheltered in the branches. For more than an hour they sat through the thunder and lightning while the rain fell in sheets. When at last the storm finished she and the chimpanzees moved back down the mountainside to a point overlooking a lake. Everything was jewelled with raindrops. The sun broke through as the storm clouds moved away. Goodall tells how she slipped into a state of heightened consciousness, one she finds impossible to render in words. She lost her sense of self and instead felt the oneness of her own life with that of the chimpanzees and the trees, the air, the earth, the sky. She was overcome by an intense awareness of colour and sound and smell. It was a mystical experience, a way of apprehending the world directly by means of the heart and soul. 'An unseen hand had drawn back a curtain,' she writes. 'In a flash of "outsight" I had known timelessness and quiet ecstasy, sensed a truth of which mainstream science is merely a small fraction.'

Albert Camus also reported a personal peak experience, albeit in a more minor key, in a notebook entry written in 1943 and dated 20 May. The fact that this is one of the very few dated entries is itself significant, and shows the value Camus placed on the experience. It was a hot, heavy evening and he was lying on the grass thinking about how he would feel if he were to die and 'for the first time,' he writes, 'a bizarre feeling of satisfaction and plenitude.'

Finally, another way of describing peak experiences is the one we met already when we looked at Bach's miraculous recovery from illness: *flow*, better known in the sporting world as *the zone*. Psychologists use these terms to describe moments when we are performing at peak efficiency, without conscious effort, and see ourselves doing things with magical grace and excellence. Daniel Goleman quotes a gold medal skier at the 1994 winter Olympics who could not remember the details of her descent, only the flow of it. 'I felt like a waterfall,' she said.

These examples give us the flavour of a peak experience. In an appendix to his book Maslow breaks down the flavour into its constituent ingredients.

🏵 *First,* people who have had a peak experience report a clear and intuitive sense that the universe is one integrated whole. Every part, including the person having the experience, is joined to every other. Conflicts move towards resolution and opposites are seen to be one.

🏵 *Second,* the experience deepens and widens perception to include everything, without question and with total acceptance. It suspends normal standards of judgement. We equally and fully perceive and give equal importance to every part of the universe.

🏵 *Third,* the experience raises us to a point where we can see things and people in the universe objectively. This amounts to a God-like view of the universe as something that has meaning in itself and doesn't just have meaning in relation to the needs of humanity or of any particular human.

🏵 *Fourth,* and at the same time as the universe is seen as objectively real, we transcend and forget the ego. Peak experiences quite literally take us out of ourselves, and negative emotions such as anxiety melt away.

🏵 *Fifth,* peak experiences don't need to be justified. We feel they are valuable in themselves, i.e. valuable because they exist and not because they lead to something else.

🏵 *Sixth,* and following on from the last point, peak experiences show us there is something in life worth living for, something that has deep value in itself. The peak experience refutes nihilism absolutely and without any further room for debate.

🏵 *Seventh,* the experience suspends notions of time and space. We may see all time at once, or feel a minute to be a lifetime, or lose any sense of being located in any particular place.

❧ *Eighth*, we feel that everything in the universe is right and good and beautiful, including things we normally think of as ugly or evil. Illness, death and cruelty form part of the pattern and we accept them as such. (This does not imply callousness to the victims of evil. Callousness is something that the separated and selfish ego feels. In the peak experience we and the victim are joined as one and raised above callousness and suffering alike.)

❧ *Ninth*, the God-like view of the universe means that we no longer feel emotions like condemnation and shock. These reactions can only exist where there is a partial and in some sense selfish view of the universe.

Maslow's tenth point is particularly interesting because it relates to his concept of certain values as intrinsic to *being*. B-values, as he called them, include such things as truth, simplicity, justice, beauty, unity, goodness, transcendence and perfection. They are the eternal truths of all spiritual traditions. During a peak experience, when we are at our most perceptive and most open, the B-values are seen as being facts about the universe. In other words, the universe *is already* true, simple, just, beautiful, unified, good, transcendent and perfect. In a peak experience this statement is not based on faith or assertion. It is the plain report of a direct perception: this is what I saw.

Further characteristics identified by Maslow include a feeling of freedom and self-determination; a sense of being more oneself, differentiated from everyone else but at the same time selfless and free of ego concerns; higher degrees of spontaneity and openness; and an ability to see and experience the sacred even in the small concerns of daily life. We hardly need to point out the clear relationship between the sense of the universe sketched out here and Bach's view of the universe as a meaningful unity.

paradigm shifts

When we think about how science has shaped our knowledge of the world we often think in terms of addition. Two hundred years ago we had fact one and fact two; a hundred years later we had fact ten and eleven as well; today we have added nineteen and twenty; tomorrow we will add twenty-one. Science is a steady accumulation of fact, each scientist labouring away to add a brick or two to the growing tower of things we know. This is the common-sense view, but it's no more than partially correct. In his book *The Structure of Scientific Revolutions* Thomas Kuhn shows how scientific breakthroughs actually happen in an entirely different way. Science is not addition but revolution. Fact one and two crumble away when our world-view changes, and are replaced by different facts. We don't add to the tower, we tear it down and start anew.

In Kuhn's view true science can't start until enough people agree where the first tower should be built. This means that in all human history up until the time of Isaac Newton there was no 'true science' of light, because there was no single accepted theory. Every researcher scratched out his own patch of ground and started a new structure based on his own theory and his own methodology and his own set of worthwhile questions. People spent their energy defining and redefining foundations. More esoteric problems – the upper floors of the tower – were never addressed. This only changed when Newton's *Opticks* presented a theory of light with enough explanatory power to convince most of the other people working in the field. With a firm base on which to build, scientists could agree for the first time on what problems needed to be addressed and on the ground rules for addressing them. This set of shared assumptions – the tower should go here and look like this – is what Kuhn means when he speaks of a *paradigm*. A paradigm is essential for real science to begin, because without a paradigm things are too fractured to hold together.

The creation of the first paradigm in an area of research is the beginning of science. The theory that possesses all the people working in an area promises to explain events in the real world. Making this promise come true by devising experiments and measuring things is the work of 'normal' science, and takes up the careers of most scientists. The paradigm tells us what to look for and what to expect, and gives us confidence and direction, leading to a depth of study that would not be possible without it. But the paradigm is never perfect. Not everything fits. Over time unexplainable phenomena accumulate. At first they can be ignored or explained away as anomalies, experimental problems, special cases, but eventually enough of them pile up to cause a crisis. The existence of a crisis causes more scientists to work on the thorny problems using more and more inventive and unusual methods and theories. Eventually one of these new ideas proves to have enough explanatory force to account for the problem data and so a new paradigm is formed. Everybody sees that the tower is the wrong shape and in the wrong place, and the bricks are taken down ready for rebuilding. The replacement of an old paradigm by a new one is *a paradigm shift* – a moment when one accepted idea of reality is replaced by a new one.

Kuhn based his model for change on the way the humanities break up art and literature into periods: classicism giving way to romanticism, modernism collapsing into post-modernism and so on. If we define a paradigm loosely as a set of beliefs it is easy to see how doctors, priests, architects and cooks all work in paradigms of one sort or another, and how the idea of the paradigm shift can be applied as much to the changing *Zeitgeist* of all humanity as to the individual consciousness of one individual. This is what Marilyn Ferguson does in her book *The Aquarian Conspiracy*. According to Ferguson we are living today in a new paradigm. In the past we saw humanity in opposition to nature. We tried to tame it and bring it under control as if it were a dangerous enemy. From our new tower we see ourselves as part of nature, sharing her capacity for endless invention and transcendence of limits.

Ferguson describes peak experiences in terms of paradigms as well. A peak experience can be a personal paradigm shift, a moment of transformation and enlargement in which we find new levels of consciousness and new ways of seeing. Once we undergo this experience it can change us for ever. We are moved to break down the walls and build afresh and the effect of this can be startling. When Saul turns into St Paul, when Siddhartha Gautama changes overnight into the Buddha, we could say we are seeing the results of permanent shifts caused by overwhelming peak experiences. But that isn't the only and may not be the best way of describing these events.

Maslow added a preface to *Religions, Values, and Peak Experiences* a few years after its first publication. Here he makes a distinction between the one-off peak experience that visits people at random and the more permanent and self-willed form of enlightenment that he names the *plateau experience*. The difference between the two is in their names. A peak is a high point between two stretches of land. A plateau is a high place that continues. We reach a peak and have nowhere to go but down. We climb to a plateau and stay at that height for the rest of our journey. Life on the plateau is more than just 'peaking' and there is always an element of application involved in reaching it – it takes time and effort. This we see in the histories of Saul and Buddha. The former trained as a rabbi at the age of fourteen and was a rigorous and committed Pharisee before his illumination; the latter passed through six years of austerity and mortification before his miraculous night. The concept of the plateau experience reminds us how a genuine paradigm shift – a permanent move to a new way of seeing like those undertaken by Saul and Buddha – follows a period spent on the slow work of normal science. We have to start building the first tower as best we can where we are. That always takes time.

beyond words

In *Heal Thyself* Bach recommended spiritual exercises such as meditation, quiet contemplation and the deliberate stilling of thought as a way to get a clearer idea of our feelings and move into a closer relationship with our spiritual selves. This echoes the many traditions that make going beyond thought a condition of reaching the heights. This is why the techniques used to create an inner shift – listening to music, fasting, deliberate isolation, meditation, chanting, ritual, dancing and prayer – are contemplative, repetitive and hypnotic. As seekers after direct experience of truth we have to abandon the rush to words and the plague of constant rationalising that goes on in our heads. We have to move to a point where we can stop thinking, allow distractions to flow past, and just be.

The need to go beyond words means that when we come back to words we are forced to use inadequate metaphors and similes to describe what we felt. The experience is too complete and simple for us fully to explain it. This is why Camus called his experience bizarre: his rational thought couldn't account for it. When they come, peak and plateau experiences are simple and direct, so simple that as soon as we write them down they seem insignificant. Indeed, Maslow suggests that trying to justify them in words immediately devalues them. The only way to understand what they are is to know them directly.

a god-sent gift

In *Ye Suffer from Yourselves* Bach made using the essences part of this spiritual tradition of direct intuitive knowing and acceptance when he described how they enable a link to a higher consciousness:

> The action of these remedies is to raise our vibrations and open up our channels for the reception of our Spiritual Self, to flood our natures with the particular virtue we need, and wash out from us the fault which is causing harm. They are able, like beautiful music,

or any gloriously uplifting thing which gives us inspiration, to raise our very natures, and bring us nearer to our Souls: and by that very act, to bring us peace, and relieve our sufferings.

By 'raising our natures' the essences open the lines of communication with our higher self, our heart, our soul, and so with the greater universe. Once the connection is made the higher consciousness can instruct us using the hushed tones of intuition and conscience. And of course this was part of how Bach found the essences in the first place, which is why Nora Weeks referred to them as 'truths undiscoverable through the intellect'.

As Kuhn showed, in the world of science the movement towards a paradigm shift takes place gradually over time. The same is true when we set out towards our own inner paradigm shift and start using the flower essences or begin quiet meditation or other spiritual exercises. The essences don't suddenly lift us into heaven; instead they increase our awareness slowly and take time to take us up the mountain. They are closer to the plateau than they are to the peak; they lead to permanent change rather than to a one-off high. Valerie Miller's account of how they worked for her is typical. Now a counsellor and psychotherapist, she started using Bach essences in 1985 after hearing a talk on them in the crypt at Worcester Cathedral.

The first two years after discovering the remedies were a revelation to me. Life took on new meaning. Old resentments, regrets, anger about the past, slowly changed into positive thoughts about the present and the future. It's hard to say at what point I realised the profound change in my outlook and attitudes to life, the change was so subtle – all I can remember is never before experiencing such a feeling of being at one with all that was around me. It was wonderful to be able to let go of all the negativity of the past and for it to no longer have any effect on me.

Bach chose the path of simplicity and quiet when he left London and began his long journey across England and Wales looking for healing plants. He based his choice on a belief that at the right level of seeing everything in nature is simple. The system of thirty-eight essences is a God-sent gift, he says, and as a gift from God it is a perfect distillation of nature. There is nothing to add and nothing to explain. If we go the other path, and try to rationalise them, account for them, theorise about them, make them a tool of our ego, discover their active element, distil them, turn them into pills with stated strengths, worry about dosage and side effects, we are moving away from a direct experience of the gift. We destroy their special value by questioning them, just as we devalue a peak experience the moment we put it into words.

making a link with nature

It will be clearer what we mean by 'a distillation of nature' if we look at how essences are made. There are two preparation systems, known as the sun method and the boiling method. Both processes are direct and straightforward.

❦ **In the sun method** we fill a clear glass bowl with clean water. The water can come from a local stream or spring or we use good quality bottled mineral water or rainwater. We pick flowers off the plant so they fall directly onto the surface of the water. Then we leave the bowl lying on the ground in full sunlight. After about three hours we remove the flower heads. We mix the energised water half-and-half with brandy, which helps preserve the water and keep it fresh. (We use a naturally made French cognac, but any strong spirit will do just as well. If you have concerns about the alcohol in the remedies, see page 230.) The resulting mix is the mother tincture.

❀ **In the boiling method** we cut six-inch lengths of new flowering twigs so they fall into a large enamel or stainless-steel pan. We add water to cover the collected plant material. We boil the pan, uncovered, and leave it to simmer for half an hour before removing it from the heat. We cover the pan and stand it out in the garden to cool. When the water has cooled we filter the liquid and mix as before half-and-half with brandy to make the mother tincture.

Weeks tells how Bach was keen to keep 'the human element' out of the process. He avoided touching the flowers when picking them – we still use scissors today – and used twigs or a blade of grass to remove flower heads from the bowl rather than use his fingers. Where holding new-cut flowers was unavoidable Weeks recommended laying a large leaf on the hand to avoid touching the blooms. Even human shadows were avoided, and at the Bach Centre we guide visitors away from bowls lying in the sun so they will not cast a shadow on them. Simple nature is the key to a successful process and not human complications. The maker of essences is a necessary agent, a servant rather than a wizard, and anybody can prepare essences, even the most out of balance. The idea that one needs to be some kind of initiate to produce good remedies is a misunderstanding.

Whichever method we use, whichever remedy we are making, the act of making remedies takes place in and with nature. Remedies are made in the morning, ideally before nine o'clock, when the day is fresh. For the sun method essences the sun must be strong and there must be no cloud, while many of the boiling method plants bloom in the early spring when the days can be bright and raw at the same time. Crouching down in the late August heat to collect gentian or standing gathering sun-coloured flowers from gorse bushes or stretching up for sprays of blossoming cherry plum we are in direct contact with nature, and also with a long tradition that sees people harvesting gifts from nature for food, clothing, medicine and religious uses. Certainly many people who make their own essences find meaning in the activity. Diana Antonaroli's experience is typical of this. A psychologist in Rome, she has used the flowers for over nine years. 'A very significant passage was when I prepared my first remedy,' she says. 'The contact with the plant was an incredible experience. I really feel the flower remedies are a bridge from earth to a superior nature where real life is, where our superior self lives.'

The majority of remedy users who don't make their own still like to dwell on the link with nature and plants. One such is Karen Briscombe, a Bach practitioner from England. 'Linking in my mind's eye to the actual plant or imagining the tree helps to establish a deeper contact with the unseen world and its powerful healing properties,' she says. 'I have always been able to relate to flower nature spirits and this is an extension of that process. It deepens the relationship and gives back my appreciation and gratitude.' Rosemary Barry from Australia agrees: 'I identify strongly with nature, observing her beauty and lessons, putting down my impressions on paper and uniting with her in ritual and ceremony. It is a constant pleasure to walk in the National Parks and in the bush and feel the energy the different flora and fauna give off. The remedies feel as familiar as nature itself.' The link remains strong because everything that happens to the mother tincture on its journey from the open countryside to the shop shelf is equally simple and straightforward. Remedies are not succussed or artificially energised or doctored in any way. 'The way they are made brings a special feel to this form of healing unlike any other,' says Claire Bickerton, who bought her first bottle of Rescue™ Remedy in 1996. 'They symbolise the gentleness of the countryside, the rolling hills and the smell of spring, in the subtle and gentle way they bring hope and relief from winter.'

the uses of simplicity

Selecting and taking essences is as simple as eating when hungry or drinking when thirsty. We just think about how we feel and take the ones we need. The process helps us focus on our emotions and make them conscious. It gives us a still space in our lives, a moment of contemplation. With this in mind many practitioners advise people to hold the essences in the mouth for a few moments before swallowing so as to give time to think about why they are being taken. This is not essential to make the remedies work – after all, they work just as well on babies, who presumably don't know they are taking them – but it helps us get closer to how we feel and how we want to feel. 'One client said that taking the remedies gave her permission to think safely and without judgement about what concerned her,' says Alison Murphy, a practitioner in the west of England. 'She felt that those moments when she was actually holding the drops on her tongue had wrought remarkable changes in her outlook and inner peace.'

As for dosage, when to take them, when to stop taking them, again simplicity is the keynote: take a few drops at a time as often as you need to, take them when you need them, stop taking them when you don't. The instructions are so simple that many people coming to flower essences for the first time are actually confused, feeling they must have missed something. Surely it can't be that easy? Where are the warnings against taking too much or getting addicted? Where are the long lists of contraindications and side effects? There are none, for the point of taking essences is to stand aside from this babble of worry and just be aware and do it.

Just being aware and just doing it is a Zen approach to development. Zen masters teach that the simplest task can be a way of enlightenment as long as every act and every moment are fully experienced. So in the *chado*, the tea ceremony, everything from greeting one's guests to boiling the water to serving the tea to bidding farewell is ritualised by the way hosts and guests pay complete attention to what they are doing. The ceremony can take four hours to complete, but because everything is invested with personal meaning these four hours are not wasted time but moments of great and intrinsic significance. According to Sir George Trevelyan, the founder of the Wrekin Trust, the coming age is one in which *every* act in life will tend to become sacred and significant, just like making tea in the tea ceremony. Thanks to a wider view – a broader paradigm of our place in the universe – we will begin to see how the small things of daily life form part of the great pattern. We will take joy from making a pair of trousers or digging the garden, as Bach did when he was at Mount Vernon and as twenty-first-century downshifters do today. Every moment we live can become a chance to acknowledge our relationship with the universe. By choosing and taking a remedy as simply as possible, 'pure as it is; free from science, free from theories', we turn the simple act of taking a flower into a significant moment of contemplation, like the *chado*, like Zen itself. Our personality has a chance to build more abundant awareness of itself and its structure, and so move towards its own personal paradigm shift.

This is the real use of simplicity.

v ❀ connecting

No man is an island entire of itself; every man is a piece of the continent, a part of the main. If a clod be washed away by the sea, Europe is the less, as well as if a promontory were, as well as if a manor of thy friend's or of thine own were. Any man's death diminishes me, because I am involved in mankind. And therefore never send to know for whom the bell tolls: it tolls for thee.

– John Donne, seventeenth-century preacher and poet

> The remedies mean a greater connection with all living things. I have been drawn to gardening, and find pleasure in creating a garden and nurturing my plants and trees. My garden responds and looks and feels greener and more lush. I enjoy giving my plants Rescue™ Remedy and Walnut when I re-plant them, and am delighted to see them settle and thrive.
>
> – Judy Beveridge

three remedies to connect

In moments of great insight we feel that all life is connected. But away from the peaks and plateaux of human experience we can feel alone and cut off from other people. The three essences in Edward Bach's group against loneliness are all concerned with interconnectedness and its lack. They help us grow out towards others more effectively so that we can avoid loneliness even when we choose to be alone.

❀ **Impatiens** enhances our appreciation of stillness and slowness so that we can give ourselves and others time to develop at whatever pace is right. People needing this flower want to do everything at top speed. They streamline their lives by avoiding friends, colleagues, family members and lovers. They become isolated, and their irritable manner doesn't encourage others to break through the barrier.

❀ **Water Violet** helps us move easily from self-reliance to interdependence. In a negative Water Violet state we have allowed enjoyment of our own thoughts and activities to turn into aloofness and reserve. The flower helps us break down these barriers so we can offer and ask for help and companionship.

❀ If people in negative Water Violet and Impatiens states seek isolation, negative **Heather** will do anything to avoid it. In this state we are so full of our own concerns that we burst to tell others about them. But we forget to listen, so that instead of building a mutual exchange of support and understanding our monologues drive people away.

stars

I was commuting several hours a day by train. My home station was a couple of miles from my house, and if I got back after seven o'clock in the evening there were no more buses and I had to walk home. I often got to the station after seven o'clock because there were always so many things to do at work and I liked to be on top of everything. I enjoyed the sense of speed and fullness – irons in the fire, I called it. And I enjoyed being at work late (and early) more than I enjoyed being at work during regular hours. The early morning and the evening were quiet times. There were few people around to interrupt my flow, few phone calls and no irrelevant chit-chat to eat up my time.

After a couple of streets and a pub the walk home went along the side of hedgerows and open fields. There were no street lights. The road ran very straight and in the winter when the dark came early I could watch the red tail-lights of the cars dwindle for whole minutes before they winked away at the corner a couple of miles away.

I would race the cars, walking fast with my head down to spy out the shadow of uneven pavement in the passing headlights. The walk home took exactly forty-two minutes if I really pushed, and I always really pushed. Then one day I stopped, just like that. I'd had enough rushing. I looked up and saw a million stars that had nothing to do with me.

discover stillness: impatiens

A few years ago there was a programme on television in which an experienced children's nanny gave advice to parents with problem kids. One mother was at her wits' end with her little boy, who would play up, scream and throw things every time she took him on a shopping trip. The camera accompanied them to the supermarket and showed mother and child in action. Sure enough he was a horror, and we could understand why Mum tried to get the whole thing over as fast as possible. She kept him strapped into the trolley and answered his questions in monosyllables so his talking wouldn't hold her up. She darted from place to place, all hair and eyes and grabbing hands, and was harassed and red in the face by the time she got through the checkout. The child was crying and the gauntlet was thrown: how would Nanny cope with this?

In a negative Impatiens state we don't give time to others. We try to do our work by ourselves so that slower people won't hold us back. If we are waiting for somebody else to do something we have to fight the temptation to grab hold of it and finish it ourselves. We are bad teachers, bad managers, bad leaders in our negative state, because delegation and tuition and guidance take too long. Although we have good intuition and higher-than-average intelligence we lack wisdom. We think so much about speed and action that we miss the details those annoying slow people pick up. If things go well and quickly we have wonderful stamina and find no task too much but our frustration at slowness can exhaust us. In a bad temper we will slam doors and kick out at irritating objects, and end up injuring ourselves. Fortunately for our health our tempers cool as quickly as they flare.

When Nanny picked up the gauntlet her answer came in the form of positive Impatiens qualities: patience with other people's needs and a willingness to be in the moment ('doing the shopping') rather than thinking only of the end of a task ('to have done the shopping'). Nanny took her time. She discussed every purchase with the little boy. Did he know what this was called? Could he reach it and put it in the trolley for her? Did he like this type of baked beans or that? The result was that the child was a delight – bright, interested, keen to learn, polite and well behaved. Nanny took ten minutes longer to do the shopping and everyone left calm and happy.

Impatiens is the flower of stillness and patience. It teaches us to appreciate the slower things in life. It gives us time to connect, time to be with our children and the people we love, time to stop and smell the flowers (and gaze at the stars and consider the beans). We can appreciate chores like ironing and washing dishes (and shopping and going from place to place) if we stop trying to get them done as fast as possible and take the time to make them fun and meaningful. The person who interrupts us and slows us down may have an insight to share that will change our lives. All it takes is a small paradigm shift, the decision to include processes and the incidental in the set of valuable experiences.

Impatiens glandulifera makes an easy-to-remember remedy because its Latin name reflects its habits and its habits reflect what it is for. It was introduced into Europe in 1913 and since 1930 has spread rapidly throughout Britain. As an annual it grows from nothing to six feet in a couple of months. It prefers riverbanks or low-lying wet ground, where its fast growth and fecundity quickly cover the ground with a jungle of tall upright plants that crowd out slower growers. The irritability and quick temper of the Impatiens person is reflected in the sharp-toothed leaves, and the plant's sense of hurry extends to the way it sheds its seeds: touching a ripe seed pod causes a small explosion that scatters seeds like shrapnel.

I am a tour operator and run my own company. My problem was a reluctance to get to grips with important jobs, plus an impatience to get everything done as quickly as possible. This may sound like a contradiction, but it meant that every day I just worked on the things I could finish quickly. More difficult tasks got left until last, and as more easy tasks cropped up all the time, so the difficult ones got left longer and longer. I tried Hornbeam and Impatiens and the effect was instant: I felt settled enough to tackle the difficult jobs and an enormous relief at finally clearing my in-tray. – Lynn Hinton

a remedy for modern times?

After teaching Bach's system of flower essences for several years I have become wary of claims that this or that flower particularly suits the modern world. I have heard students declare that more people than ever before need Agrimony because we are all so conscious of the need to appear cheerful and hide our feelings. I have heard similar claims made for Mimulus because of all the food scares, nuclear weapons, wars and bad news. Other people promote Walnut as the main modern remedy – just look at all the changes in our lives and the way we are bombarded with outside influences. Why, the average Briton is subjected to more than a thousand commercial messages every week....

Living in interesting times makes us feel special and important, so it's tempting to believe that our lives are uniquely complex and that things were simpler in the past. But if we look past our prejudices we soon see how the same challenges and out-of-balance emotions have existed at all stages of history. In the past wives, servants, slaves and courtiers would have been well advised to hide their feelings and pretend to be happy. Native Americans in the north and the south of that continent had changes and outside influences to deal with that make computerisation and advertising look like footnotes, as did European peasants affected by enclosure and the Industrial Revolution. The billions who lived through civil and international war or at times of religious or political intolerance must have needed all the quiet courage they could muster to face the named and concrete fears that rose up to threaten them.

Knowing this, I will not make my own case for a quintessential modern remedy. I'm sure that if I did my choice could be criticised in exactly the same way. But if I *were* to yield to the temptation (and I won't) I would select Impatiens as the main flower for our current lifestyle, and indeed for our lifestyle over much of recent history.

Since the Industrial Revolution the West has prized efficiency and productivity above other values, and has exported this bias to all parts of the world along with its machine tools and assembly plants. We measure efficiency and productivity by counting things, and the habit has stuck to such an extent that we now treat all the things we can count as commodities. This is how flesh and red-blooded men and women end up as hands or headcount or units of labour or human resources. This is how time – our precious life on the planet – becomes money. Much of modern technology achieves value by saving time (which explains the computer's success as a product) and because of its economic value we favour those uses of time that have focused and practical outcomes. Problem solving – the kind of intelligence that can do crosswords and calculate interest payments – is clearly practical. Learning facts and skills is practical as well. But contemplation and meditation are less obviously useful. They don't make wealth so they aren't worth much.

As the writer Guy Claxton points out in *Hare Brain Tortoise Mind*, we are wrong to undervalue contemplative states. Einstein was renowned for spending large amounts of time doing nothing and gazing at nothing. Many artists and writers are the same, and spend as much time looking at the ceiling or at the clouds as they do actually painting or writing. Religions of all types stress the value of withdrawing from logical thought and spending time in contemplation. Slow thinking – tortoise thinking, in Claxton's phrase – is the wellspring of creativity and wisdom. Indeed, research shows that when our employers and teachers try to get us to speed up the things we do – whether by offering us rewards or threatening us with punishment, or even just saying, 'Couldn't you do that faster?' – we respond by doing things less well and less creatively.

Perhaps we all need to think about Impatiens and about the need to slow down and stop, so as to rediscover ourselves and the wisdom that we overlook in our drive for results today, now, if not yesterday. But I must declare an interest here, for it may have led to favouritism. Impatiens is my type remedy. My challenge in life is to learn patience and the utter difference between living fast and living. I'm still working on it. Fortunately I have time.

reach out: water violet

Hottonia palustris is a still, upright and particular plant. It only grows in pools, ditches and still streams, often some way away from firm land. Nora Weeks recommended using a crook-handled walking stick to pull the plants towards the bank so as to gather the flowers without getting wet. Water violet keeps its feathery leaves out of sight under the water, at the base of a long erect stem, where they help to keep the plant upright. At the very top of the stem the small flowers appear in a cluster.

The positive qualities of Water Violet include self-reliance and a sense of self-worth, coupled with a certain aristocratic choosiness about living conditions. Water Violet people like time to themselves to enjoy their own company and their own pursuits, and they naturally grow up towards the stars rather than out towards others. Their few select friends are their roots, their hidden base of leaves that helps them grow their own way. In return balanced Water Violet people can offer valuable support when they judge it is right to do so, for they are thoughtful, capable and intelligent.

The negative Water Violet state starts when the positives outgrow themselves and move into the extreme. The Water Violet person so far removes herself from others that she can no longer connect. At the negative extreme of Water Violet we find isolation, aloofness and separation. Other people consider us proud and turn away, while we in turn find it hard to unbend. We are social animals, whether or not we think so, and for all social animals separation is a killer. It robs us of our sense of identity because we can no longer define ourselves by our relationship with others. It leaves us more open to depression and loss of will and purpose.

Part of growing is turning selfishness to selflessness. The way to higher growth is through involvement with the world rather than withdrawal from it. We are here to climb through, not turn away. This demands that we learn to empathise with the pain and suffering in other lives. If we don't do this we will not make use of our gifts and so not develop fully. We can't help others if they no longer approach us. Water Violet can help us reconnect ourselves to the wider world, anchoring our roots into the soil so that we can grow.

In general I am quiet, though not shy. Throughout my whole life I alternated time spent socialising with hours spent alone walking the dog, cycling, thinking and reading. I love other people but get easily worn by loud and overly assertive types. I remember as a child feeling different, and aware of undercurrents beneath the surface of life. I looked on many of my contemporaries as giggly and shallow and tended to keep apart. – M.M.

I suffered great loneliness when my husband left. I was too proud to ask friends to go out to the theatre with me – I would rather not go than seem to need company. I built a real barrier around myself and found it impossible to reach out to others. Now I am able to enjoy the company of friends and working colleagues whilst retaining my need for privacy. – Lynne Langley

wood

She was a large lady and lived down our street. She wore a tightly buttoned tweed coat even in summer, and was aged around fifty. She had crooked teeth, a reddish complexion and two black eyes as bright and direct as a bird's.

I admit I used to avoid her. If I saw her when I was crossing the park and she was walking in the same direction I would slow down so as not to catch her up. If I saw her coming towards me I would veer off the path with a quick wave and a smile (still out of earshot) and head over to the far exit. It was quicker to go the long way round than to risk the 'hello' that would uncork the monologue.

Sometimes neither was possible. Lost in thought, I was already level with her, or she had fixed me like a worm with her eye and I was too close to make a switch to the second path plausible. Or she might be passing at the very moment I opened the door to leave the house in the morning or standing just around the street corner as I turned it and stopped to avoid knocking her down. Then I would be trapped.

Her conversation was a series of statements. She asked no questions and left no room for me to insert an oar and challenge the flood. I heard about her hospital appointments and what she said and what the doctor said and what she said to what the doctor said. Without pause or obvious link she moved on to the doings of relatives and friends, as far as these concerned her, and their names bobbed briefly to the surface never to return. No space to ask who was who, because she was already talking about the weather and its effect on her garden and the state of the street outside her house now that the council... and the contents of last night's television broadcast, never the same since....

I would find myself backing away or edging past, nodding and smiling and with an apologetic dip of the shoulder and wave of the hand. And she would follow, her face turned to me like a great vacant searchlight, her eyes unfocused or focused inside, calling me back and seeming not to notice my grimace or my shuffling.

Then one day we lost our central heating. It was the day before Christmas. My wife mentioned it to a neighbour in passing – we were waiting for the plumber – and a few minutes later there was a knock on the door.

It was her. She'd talked to our neighbour and didn't like to think of us in a cold house over Christmas. She knew somebody who chopped logs for a living. He had a whole shed full of wood. She took me round there and thanks to her negotiation the man gave me a barrow-load of logs for our open fire, free of charge. She left while I was loading the barrow. The log man closed the door after her. 'That's typical of her,' he said. 'She's one in a million.'

listen: heather

In *Thus Spake Zarathustra*, the German philosopher Friedrich Nietzsche claimed that the greatest thing a human being can experience is complete self-contempt. What he meant by 'self-contempt' was the ability to escape from everyday concerns, riddled as they are with self and self-interest, and ascend into a realm of selflessness in which our personal identity merges with the wholeness of the universe. This is the height towards which the positive Heather person ascends. Indeed, the discovery of the remedy was linked at the outset to that movement from the narrow self to the wide universe. This is how Edward Bach told the story:

> 'I got up and went straight to a woman I knew about, self-centred and utterly worldly, and I said to her, "What do you think is the most beautiful sight in the world? Have you ever seen anything that makes you think it possible that there is a God? " Without the least hesitation she replied, "Yes, the mountains covered with heather. "'

We need the Heather flower when we become so absorbed in our self and our material lives that we lose the ability to hear the problems of others and instead talk only about our own. We are the pub bore in a Heather state, hemming people in a corner and blocking their escape while we tell our interminable anecdotes. We are 'buttonholers' and needy children, holding on to the lapels of our listeners to stop them getting away, following them down the street, desperately sucking up the energy of their presence while barely noticing them as individuals. Being alone and unheard causes us great anguish and fear so we attach ourselves to anyone, with no pride or guile. And while we fear losing our audience, other people shun us because we are so tiring to be with. They see us as traps to be avoided.

The Heather remedy incarnates gentleness, silence, service and connection with causes greater than our own. An easy and sociable talker, Heather also listens to and understands the troubles of others. She is free from petty concerns and absorbed in the life and struggle of other people and of humanity as a whole. She is able to draw on her bad experiences so as to empathise with the experiences of others. She has learned to measure her troubles and find them small compared with the troubles of the world, so that she is truly unselfish and a great friend to those in need. Taking Heather when we are trapped in our world of words helps us reconnect and move back towards this higher point of balance.

Heather is one of the least-used remedies, perhaps because none of us wants to think we need it. Though strangely, like me with the wood lady, we are quick to see it in others. Perhaps we should be slower to jump and quicker to listen.

stardust

According to current thinking none of the complex atoms existed when the universe began. Only the simplest – hydrogen and helium and a trace of lithium – came into being along with the big bang. In a short essay called 'Can Science Answer Every Question?' the astrophysicist Martin Rees discusses where the rest of the elements come from. His answer is: stars.

A star starts out as a giant ball of about seventy-five per cent hydrogen and twenty-five per cent helium, held in place by gravity. Hydrogen is the simplest of atoms, with just one proton in its nucleus and one electron orbiting it. Gravity pulls the gas in towards the centre. As the atoms of hydrogen get closer together they heat up, and when the centre of the star is hot enough and the atoms are close enough together the protons in individual atoms smash into each other with such force that they start to fuse. Fusion makes the stars shine. The same process powers nuclear fusion bombs, but in the star the massive amount of energy released by fusion is controlled by gravity so that it is gradual and even rather than sudden and explosive.

When the simple hydrogen atoms fuse together they create more of the heavier element helium. Eventually a star will fuse all the hydrogen at its core into helium. As it does so the core gets denser so that its gravity and temperature increase further. When the core is dense enough it starts to pull some of the helium atoms together with enough force to make them fuse as well. In this way stars gradually work their way up through the periodic table. At each stage a core amount of the preceding atom fuses to produce new elements. A star ends up layered like an onion, with traces of the simpler atoms towards the outside and the last-created complex atoms towards its heart. Among the atoms produced in the star are oxygen and carbon, which are the basis of life on earth.

Our own star, the sun, is too small to go much further than carbon. But when a very big star has used up all its potential fuel it can collapse and trigger off a huge explosion, a supernova, that blasts the onion skins apart and spreads atoms – including the heavier atoms such as gold and platinum, formed in the collapse – around the universe. Eventually some of this debris will be involved in the creation of new suns and, sometimes, new solar systems with planets like ours. Way back at the birth of our solar system this is what happened: dust from ancient stars came together at the creation of a new star, and some of this dust ended up as the planet Earth and went into creating our bodies and everything else alive or not that we can see around us.

Astrophysicists like Rees view the universe as a single incredibly vast inter-connected system: 'we are all one' is not an article of faith but a statement of fact. We must abandon the Romantic idea of the single solitary individual, separated from other people and from the natural universe. We can't be separate because we are made of the same stuff. Every atom of carbon in us, every trace of iron in our blood, even the air our bodies burn and the rings we exchange when we marry, all this comes from the stars. You and I and the people we avoid and snub and ignore every day are the same stuff and share the same inheritance. A billion stars are our collective ancestors, and when our bodies die and our solar system fades to a white smudge in infinity a billion stars will be our future.

6 ❀ towards intuition

inner guidance

We have seen how intuition was the key to many of Edward Bach's achievements. It enabled the apparently magical things he accomplished, from finding remedies to foretelling storms and forestalling suicides. 'He followed the thought that came first into his mind and acted upon it before reason could step in,' Nora Weeks tells us. For Bach being intuitive meant guarding against the opinions and ideas of other people and cultivating spontaneity and naturalness. It meant doing whatever seemed right at the time, without second thinking or trying to rationalise too much. 'What is called intuition,' he wrote to a friend, 'is nothing more or less than being natural, and following your own desire absolutely.'

For Bach, intuition was the voice of the higher self. When our personality is in balance the higher self guides us and shows us which way to go. As he said, 'Our souls will guide us, if we will only listen, in every circumstance, every difficulty; and the mind and body so directed will pass through life radiating happiness and perfect health, as free from all cares and responsibilities as the small trusting child.'

If we will only listen ... but listening is not always easy. Our personalities – our thought-riddled separated egos – become more insistent and persuasive as they get more out of balance. We can always find reasons for going against the soul's quiet hints. We are practised at dressing up our second thoughts as spontaneity, our rationalisations as common sense. By relaxing into who we are, by trying to see the world with fresh eyes and by the use of simple meditation techniques,

Bach says, we can again begin to hear the small voice of wisdom that can help guide us through life. Or we can use the essences, for they too are there to help. When we can't hear the voice of intuition clearly, when our personalities are too far away from our souls to hear and too full of themselves to listen, that is the time to turn aside and take the flower we need.

formalising intuition

Orthodox and complementary practitioners value intuition as one of their most important skills, an essential tool that allows them to empathise with clients and so help them more effectively. This is certainly true of flower essence practitioners. We are aware of the emphasis Bach placed on simplicity and see his intuitive approach as an example to follow. When we select essences for somebody we use all our senses, including the sixth, to help that person understand and express how she feels. Hunches and instinct, the still voice of our own higher selves, can help us select the right essences for where she is now, and help her explore why she needs them and what she wants from taking them. It's a commonplace among practitioners that before we can help other people with remedies we need to know how to help ourselves: practitioners who never use the remedies can so easily lose touch with their intuition and begin listening to their egos instead.

Awareness of Bach's own intuitive methods has led some remedy users to go a step further and formalise intuition into the creation of purely intuitive selection methods. These new practices attempt to bypass consciousness and select essences directly. They claim to simplify still further the selection of essences because we can choose them without knowing what they are for and without having to understand or be aware of how we or our clients feel. The techniques used vary from mechanical methods – using some tool as an aid to selection – to the use of intuition alone, without reference to any tool or any form of conscious thought.

Perhaps the best-known mechanical selection technique for flower remedies is dowsing. Traditional dowsers used a forked hazel twig to search for water or lost objects or patterns of energy in the earth. This is an ancient art. In all probability Moses was doing something like this when he used a divining rod to find water during the long desert march to the Promised Land, and many less famous people down through the ages have dowsed for wells and hidden springs with great success. More recently dowsers have experimented with rods made of other woods, and metal, and even nylon. But the dowsing tool most associated with selecting flower essences is the pendulum.

A pendulum is basically a weight on a string. The weight can be almost anything. Many dowsers use a crystal, but ceramic, metal, wood and glass can serve just as well. Practitioners using a pendulum to select essences might hold it over a set of stock bottles, one by one, and watch the way it swings over the different remedies. Or they might ask questions out loud such as, 'Does the remedy I need begin with the letters a, b or c?' or, 'Do I need a fear remedy?' A clockwise spin might mean 'yes' and a counter-clockwise spin 'no'; but there are no hard and fast rules for interpreting the movements of a pendulum and different practitioners work to different criteria.

A second purely intuitive technique relies on the use of specially made cards, about the size of tarot cards, each one bearing a colour picture of one of the remedy flowers. A practitioner of this method will lay out all the cards face up on the table and invite her client to select any that particularly appeal to him. (I have heard that a lot of clients seem to select Wild Rose, probably the prettiest of the remedy flowers.) Alternatively she may present them face down or in a pack, or combine them with a pendulum whose swings say 'yes' or 'no' to each one. A third device is to rack the remedy bottles into a box in such a way that the labels saying which is which can't be seen and ask the client to pick out any that she feels drawn to. Other practitioners invite their clients to touch or hold bottles and say which ones feel particularly warm; the client will end up taking those she picks.

Finally, there is the completely intuitive practitioner. This is the person who says that she only has to touch somebody or look at a client to have the right remedies pop into her head at once. For this practitioner there is no need for further debate or analysis because she *knows*. In one way this extreme – intuition that claims not to need an external prop such as a picture card or pendulum – actually completes the circle and begins again to be more like the classic consultation approach. We have already said that even the most rigorously classical practitioner of course and necessarily and without exception relies partly on intuition when selecting remedies. Nevertheless, there are a number of objections to making intuition the sole focus of selecting essences, and they apply as much to the 'I-just-know-it' people as to the more obvious dowsers and layers-out of cards.

sharing knowledge

The first objection comes from those practitioners who stress the self-help aspect of taking Bach remedies. The simplicity of the system makes it possible for anybody to use it – as with making essences, choosing them is not the preserve of experts and initiates – and Bach held this up as one of its main advantages. Practitioners who follow this line aim to share their knowledge with their clients. They find this easier to do if they describe the essences in terms of ordinary everyday emotions. Any talk of special gifts (such as being able to know somebody's innermost feelings just by looking at him or touching his arm) or of special techniques (you have to learn to dowse or meditate or contact your inner child first) can only make the remedies seem more complex than they need to be and so discourage people from using them for themselves. Many clients of dowsers remain clients indefinitely because they feel they can't learn to dowse. Seen in this light we see how the purely intuitive selectors move away from being classic Bach practitioners, concerned to share a simple technique with everyone, and instead take up the position of therapists. The therapist believes that any approach that has a positive effect on health should be embraced regardless of its difficulty or exclusivity. The practitioner believes that in the long term the only way a client will get the maximum benefit from the essences is to use them for herself.

We will suggest reasons for this belief later in this chapter. In the meantime we might take a moment to look at the Code of Practice issued by the Dr Edward Bach Foundation, as this best represents the position of the classic Bach practitioner. Bach Foundation Registered Practitioners sign up to a number of statements that make clear the importance of the conversational approach to selection. They promise to 'act as facilitators and guides'. They promise to teach their clients 'so that they can use [the system] unaided'. And clause 5.2 of the Code specifies clearly the selection method that should be used: 'When working with the 38 remedies practitioners shall always and only use the simple selection and consultation methods outlined by Dr Bach in *The Twelve Healers and Other Remedies* and shall not recommend, refer to or use any other selection methods, aids or tools.'

The practitioner's approach as set out in the Foundation's Code is *to empower people as much as possible*, as opposed to the purely therapeutic approach that aims to *cure clients as well as possible*. Good therapists see their clients again and again, because whenever the client has a problem she will return for more help. Good practitioners turn their clients free, and expect and hope to see them less and less frequently. (I should stress that this distinction is not a criticism of the work done by therapists. Many therapies demand years of study and training and hard-won expertise. Others can only be carried out effectively by a third person. Some can even be dangerous in the hands of novices. We expect clients to return to their homoeopaths, dentists, physio-therapists and massage therapists when they need more help, and we wouldn't think much of an acupuncturist who handed us a pack of needles and a chart and told us only to come back if we have problems. The practitioner's approach – encouraging *self*-help – only becomes possible with simple and safe systems like Bach.)

the comfort of clients

The classic consultation process is an open invitation to a client to discuss how he feels in his own words and in his own time. Beyond its educational value there is intrinsic benefit to be gained from this approach. Only rarely do we get permission to talk freely about our emotions. When a practitioner listens attentively it can be a wonder-fully liberating experience for a client, one that is therapeutic in itself. But like technological medicine, which helps make the hospital ward a place we fear and respect in equal measure, the more esoteric selec-tion methods can turn clients off and turn them away. Some people feel unheard and confused among the new age trappings of pendu-lums and picture cards, just as they do among the bleeps and read-outs of the modern hospital. Not liking the selection method leads them to dismiss the essences themselves as so much mumbo-jumbo. We may consider these clients need Beech, but unless we find a way to convince them that Beech is worth taking we won't reach them. And the client is justified in his scepticism when a poorly used or plain poor selection method leads to a situation where the chosen essences just don't work.

Away from the esoteric, another branch of alternative diagnostics mimics the scientific objectivity of blood tests and the CAT scan. These too can be less than satisfactory, and for the same fundamental reason. When Catherine went to see a kinesiologist and underwent muscle testing it was because she was already receiving orthodox cancer therapy and hoped to supplement that with a kinder, more complementary form of treatment. What she found was more of the same. 'The emphasis was solely on the body,' she says. 'The practitioner spent very little time talking to me and left me feeling vulnerable and lonely. The session gave the therapist information he needed to supply my body with its dietary and supplement needs but no mention was made of other needs.'

Most practitioners go cold at the idea of selecting Bach remedies in a wordless space that looks away from the person and towards some external symptom of distress. Flower essences are about expressing and understanding our emotions and feelings, our inner thoughts and dreams. We can't and shouldn't reduce them to the level of muscle tests and tick boxes. Certainly this is the conclusion Helga Braun came to when she first considered using the remedies in her practice. A veterinary doctor working in Germany, she is also qualified in reso-nance therapy and acupuncture. When it came to selecting remedies, 'resonance testing worked too, but meant reducing my patients to a pile of test sheets, which was exactly what I didn't want and was the main reason for starting to use complementary methods in the first place.' Her conclusion was the one reached by many other therapists and practitioners before and since: 'Bach was a system in its own right, to be used alone or alongside other methods.'

what guides?

These objections relate to the way professional practitioners use Bach's essences to help others. They are less relevant if we only want to help ourselves. That granted, is there a problem with using pure intuition to select the essences we personally need? If we feel we can select the right flower by picking cards or dowsing or allowing our intuition to pop its name into our head why not just do it and see what happens?

One argument against using intuitive selection to pick remedies for ourselves is that hardly any of us are *only* interested in ourselves. (If we are there are remedies for this too.) We may start using flower essences for our personal growth but sooner or later we end up suggesting them to friends, lovers, family members and work-mates. When we do we face the same dilemma as every practitioner: do I help this person to help himself, or do I take on the therapist's role? And if we choose the practitioner approach we are in the practitioner's position of realising that the easiest and most natural way to talk about and explain the remedies is that we take Mimulus when we feel afraid about something and Gentian to get over a setback. If all our experience to that point is with dowsing we will find it difficult to change our approach when we want to help a friend talk about his troubles.

A second argument is that we might only be fooling ourselves. It's all too easy to receive impulses from our lower self and assume they are the spontaneous insights of our higher self. The sick ego is very good at dressing up self-promotion and vanity and calling it insight. Maybe what we think is inner guidance is in fact ego-directed self-interest. Maybe we are using divine inspiration to excuse the selection of essences that make us look good or give us an excuse to act out our fantasies, rather than the less attractive remedies we actually need. I have always been struck by the number of remedy users who describe themselves as Vervain or Water Violet or Agrimony people and how few admit to being dyed-in-the-wool Heathers and Beeches. This is the case even when any third person can clearly see how Heather and Beech apply. Perhaps the most negative Vervain characteristics appear 'sexy' in a movie-star anti-hero kind of way – fanatical, extreme, never switching off and so on. Hollywood seldom makes action blockbusters about people who can't stop talking about themselves.

short cuts and wisdom

We come now to the third and most important argument.

Muriel Spark's eponymous heroine in *The Prime of Miss Jean Brodie* defines education as 'a leading out of what is already there in the pupil's soul'. Bach would have accepted this definition. For him, all the qualities were already latent in some part of us but had not yet been led out into the everyday light of the personality. 'Within ourselves lies all truth,' he wrote. 'We need seek no advice, no teaching but from within.' Leading out *means* making conscious. Intuitive selection fails to make conscious because *it does not oblige us to think about how we feel.* Dowsing and drawing cards may sometimes select the right flower and so restore emotional balance but that is all they do. Taking remedies becomes an end in itself. It may even hide from us how we feel, where we have gone wrong, because instead of being present in ourselves and identifying our feelings and where they come from we can use a remedy to prop ourselves up without even knowing why we need to take it. We reduce the whole system to the level of Rescue™ Remedy – quick fixes with no need for knowledge.

At first sight this objection may appear paradoxical. We have already said that the deepest insight and knowledge, the moments that Abraham Maslow called peak experiences, come in a space outside language and rational thought. And Bach spoke of doing the one right thing, without reflection, and that this was the way to be guided aright. If it is true that we can only understand our place in the universe by putting the thought-riddled personality on hold, why bring that same personality back onto centre-stage when it comes to selecting remedies? Why make selecting essences a matter of conscious thought and reflection?

There are two answers to the paradox.

❀ First, **the reason we need an essence is that we are having trouble hearing our higher selves.** The role of intuition as Bach explained it was to be a means of communication between the higher self and the personality, one that would help the personality find its right path. To be perfectly intuitive we have to be in direct communication with our higher self. Achieving intuition is therefore an aim of taking essences rather than a means of selecting them. Relying on pure intuition to select remedies for ourselves is like sending an e-mail to ask when the network will be back up, or using a broken telephone to call the phone company, or deciding to drive 500 miles to the petrol station because we have no petrol left in the tank.

❀ Second, **taking an essence helps us learn a lesson, but learning a lesson is more than taking an essence.** Every negative feeling is a hurdle to overcome and an opportunity to express a positive quality within us. Expressing that quality allows us to learn and grow. Getting past an obstacle quickly isn't necessarily the best way to learn about its nature or the best way to express a quality, especially if getting past involves walking around or taking a short cut. Often slow overcoming is the most important part of a lesson, and slow overcoming means becoming fully conscious of and understanding our negative side, step by step, taking the time that it takes. The greased ease of intuitive techniques reduces our chance of doing that simple thing.

Selecting and using flower essences in the classical way gets to better balance via the road of greater self-knowledge. We learn about our feelings first, and only then start to change them for the better. This process moves us – the lock, stock and barrel of us, the whole person – towards the kind of spontaneous intuitive living that Bach believed in. The situation is very different if we rely on a pendulum or running our hand along a row of bottles to go straight to a remedy. We are presupposing that the intuitive link with the higher self is already in place rather than being an aspiration that the essences help us attain. And if our intuition works despite everything – if the broken phone gets a signal – we get the flower without the knowledge. It's as if someone has put something in our coffee and sorted us out without telling us. The whole point of the negative emotion, which was to give us an area in which to grow and learn, is lost. Our personality is in the same position as a schoolgirl who gets her mother to do her homework. We get the right answers but have no idea what the question meant.

At an extreme, intuitive selection has us zapping the hurdles before they appear, one by one, minute by minute, so fast that we never get to climb them. We are like spinning tops, nudged back vertical at every incipient wobble and because of this all the more unstable and all the more likely to wobble again in a minute's time. We never have the space to be unaided and in balance if the only thing shoring us up is the constant finger prod of new-selected essences. The classic method of conscious reflection, on the other hand, allows us the space we need. 'Learning to use the remedies has helped me get to know myself better,' says one newly registered practitioner in England, Florence Salooja. 'I have had to look at myself objectively, and some of the things I have learned have really surprised me.' Another, Andrea Allardyce, agrees. 'You have to confront and analyse how you are feeling in order to make a selection,' she says. 'I found this very helpful in understanding myself and what type of person I am: my weaknesses, areas that need improvement, as well as my strengths.'

When we look back at Bach's own career it's striking how this deeply intuitive man took years of struggle and effort to create his system. He used his intuition wherever he could, and it guided him more and more. But he still had to walk every step of his path and make many mistakes along the way. When he helped select remedies for other people he used the classic process of sitting, and listening, and teaching. Above all he took time. There were no short cuts for him, and there are none for us. Learning takes time and life takes time, as any truly enlightened person from Buddha to St Paul knows. And now we see a further meaning behind Bach's statement in *The Twelve Healers*, that we will get most from the system if we use it in the simple and pure way in which he presented it. As well as being an everyday ritual and a link to nature, using the remedies for ourselves in the most simple kitchen cabinet way helps us learn about who we are. We can cultivate the flower within us, to its fullest possible bloom.

The need to value the process of learning suggests that attempts to create diagnostic machines are misguided, as is reliance on questionnaires or any other form of closed system that might speed up the selection process. It also accounts for the fact that the easy 'cures' achieved with intuitive selection methods often unravel just as quickly. Even if we check our reference book to find out what Larch is for after the pendulum tells us we need to take it, we still haven't taken any time as a personality to acknowledge or experience our Larch state or consider what lesson it might have for us. 'I found the pendulum would go deep but miss out important layers of the onion and important steps on the healing path,' says Rixt Spierings, a New Zealander who experimented with and abandoned dowsing and now teaches the classic method. 'I started to notice that I would get some-where (let's say another space) but not know why. I would come back to nearly square one.'

Speed and progress are not the same thing. Removing self-aware-ness from the selection process makes Bach's simple system even simpler, but the price is that it leaves out the main aim of using the essences in the first place. It sacrifices power and effectiveness and allows us to go on being blind. Simplicity becomes over-simplification, or simplism, and simplistic solutions are always based on ignorance. We should bear this in mind, for later in this book we will find more good reasons for going slowly.

self-awareness

We have seen how negative emotions give us a chance to learn and grow. But before we can learn from our feelings we have to learn how to feel. For some of us this already presents a grave difficulty.

The Harvard psychiatrist Peter Sifneos first used the term *alexithymia* in 1972. The word is compounded from the Greek words *a* (without), *lexis* (speech) and *thumos* (soul), so that if we suffer from alexithymia we have no words for what is in our soul. 'I feel bad,' we say, but can't go further and say whether 'bad' means fear, anger, depression or whatever. As a clinical condition alexithymia is a rare and sometimes crippling problem that falls outside the scope of this book; a cure may involve in-depth therapy and professional help. But in a more general sense all of us can become borderline alexithymics when conflicting unconscious moods and needs leave us marooned on our island of rationality and groping to understand our uncharted depths. The teenager awash with unnamed feelings and the working father struggling to define and communicate his need for affection can both be victims of a form of wordlessness that follows the same pattern as full-blown alexithymia.

Alexithymia makes us helpless. If we could become aware that 'bad' meant angry or sad then we could do something to clear the emotion, whether that meant meditating or watching a comedy video or taking the right flower essence. But undiagnosed emotions don't dissipate. They simmer below the surface and influence our reaction to subsequent events. Feeling depressed or irritated already and unable to do anything about it, we tend to see more and more reasons to feel that way, so that our negative states deepen.

The core to any solution is to make time for emotions. Psychologists researching mood sometimes issue test subjects with alarms that go off every few hours, and ask them to take a few minutes to think about how they feel every time the bell rings or the bleeper bleeps. This would be a bit extreme in everyday life – the alarm might itself cause quite a lot of irritation – but the principle of building thinking times into the day is a good one. We all have habits, whether listening to the radio over breakfast or singing in the shower. Breaking these habits from time to time opens up quiet spaces. We can use this time to reflect on ourselves. We may even find it helpful to write down how we feel. This has the added advantage of requiring the use of words, very much a conscious function of the mind and one that helps bring emotions into the clearest possible focus. Naming and having a feeling about an emotion immediately gives us an option to choose to feel another way. We might want to keep a journal of our feelings, or only write things down when we feel particularly bad or particularly good. And here are some other ways to think more about emotions and moods:

🌼 *We could* talk more about our feelings with our friends and partners.

🌼 *We could* stop every time we think badly about somebody – it could be somebody holding us up in a queue or a drunk or whatever – and imagine how we would feel if we were that person. (We can do the same thing with characters in soap operas and films or, even better, think back to occasions in the past where other people seemed unreasonable and incomprehensible. How did they really feel?)

🌼 *We could* go through the essences in *Bloom* and think back to times in the past when we were in that state, even if we aren't now.

Whatever route we choose to greater self-awareness the important thing is to be as specific as possible. If we feel angry we need to say exactly what kind of anger it is, such as hostility (defining somebody as the enemy and wanting to attack) or impatience (wishing they would get out of the way) or irritation (being annoyed by the things they do). A thesaurus lists lots of different kinds of anger, all subtly different. If we feel afraid, what is the trigger for our fear: personal safety, or somebody else's situation? Is it vague or specific? Is it depressed and introverted or mixed with a need to do something fast?

Naming our emotions allows us to understand and direct them so that we avoid hurting ourselves and others. And as we get better at understanding our feelings – and use the flowers to transmute them into a positive state – we find that we are better able to understand our relationships, so that the negative emotions of others will throw us off course less often. 'Relations with my family didn't change when I started taking remedies,' says Debbie Henderson, who runs a holistic health clinic in Canada, 'but my reaction to these relations changed. Things felt lighter and smoother. I was seeing a therapist at the time and she remarked how she noticed a change in me. I seemed more relaxed and less anxious.' Being more relaxed and less anxious means we can contribute more to the emotional health of the people around us. Understanding, empathy and compassion go together, and the beginning of these must be self-understanding and self-awareness – choosing to see and see below the patterns in our own hearts.

vi ✿ positivity

Love seeketh not itself to please,
Nor for itself hath any care,
But for another gives its ease,
And builds a heaven in hell's despair.
– William Blake, eighteenth-century poet, artist and engraver

I almost feel thankful, odd as that may sound, for the adversity in my life. It helped me fully appreciate what I have learned along the way, and appreciate being able to help other people, and my present fulfilling way of life. – Lynn Hall

eight positive charges

Appropriate sadness can be a positive emotion. It turns us away from pleasure and diversion and puts us into a reflective mood. It gives us time to come to terms with losses or plan how to overcome reversals and in this way actually helps us move forward. But any sadness that is more than mild quickly turns into a negative. Instead of being a springboard on which we pause and start again sadness becomes a swamp that clings and closes off and stops us moving forward. When we need help to extricate ourselves the eight essences in Edward Bach's group against despondency and despair can be a guide out of the mire. They help us use our dark feelings in the most positive way, and pass through depression instead of sinking into it.

❀ **Sweet Chestnut** helps us find hope and a sense of peace when all is darkness. Users particularly associate it with the extreme despair of bereavement and terminal illness.

❀ **Star of Bethlehem** is known as the comforter of sorrows. It helps us release trauma and shock. People often use it when they have suffered ill treatment or a bereavement.

❀ **Crab Apple** helps us accept ourselves as we are. It gives us the ability to judge the relative importance or unimportance of different aspects of our lives so that we don't become despondent over small things that don't really matter.

❀ **Willow** is about generosity, the ability to feel pleasure at the success of others even if we ourselves have been unlucky. Willow helps when we feel inclined towards self-pity and resentment.

❀ The positive characteristics of **Oak** are strength, endurance, reliability and a slow, determined and methodical approach to life. When we take these qualities to an extreme they become negatives: we think our strength inexhaustible and plod on until we break. The Oak essence picks us up when exhausted and tempers resilience with self-awareness.

❀ **Elm** is about the self-belief needed to cope with high levels of responsibility. It helps when we have so many demands on our time that we begin to doubt if anybody could manage. We agonise over letting people down and fall into despondency.

❀ **Larch** gives us that hopeful positivity that tells us we can do things as well as anybody else, and that if we try and fail that too is a way to succeed.

❀ The positive qualities of **Pine** centre around our ability to judge our actions fairly and not dwell on our mistakes. We use this flower when we feel inclined to blame ourselves and do ourselves down every time something goes wrong.

find hope: sweet chestnut

When people we love are dying or we are facing some irreducible and terrible fact such as terminal illness or extreme poverty, joy can seem like a nonsense, no more than a faraway rumour. But even in the deepest gutter there are windows on the stars. Situations that seem sure to lead to despair can instead lead to wonderful acts of courage and understanding, moments in which ordinary people rise to the heights of heroism. Sufferers can grow in ways that leave the rest of us – the lucky ones who have never had to face true despair – open-mouthed with respect and admiration.

Only people who have been through the Sweet Chestnut state can really understand it. And with their understanding they can offer comfort and support to others when they too have to come to terms with something with which it seems impossible to come to terms. I have one person in mind as I write this, not a famous person, who came through an experience among the most awful that anybody can imagine. Thinking about the bright, positive, loving light she is now to so many others I am forced to the conclusion that suffering can be a kind of blessing. Not a facile shrug of the shoulders and a trite 'it's all for the best', but a hard blessing, a way of stones, tears and terrible agony. I feel unqualified to write about it properly or do it justice. And I am weak enough to hope that I never will be so qualified. Yet if I do have to walk that path I have the comfort of knowing that I will not be alone and will not have been the first.

The quality of Sweet Chestnut's despair is completely different from that other state of despair for which Bach recommended the Gorse remedy. In a Gorse state we adopt a pessimistic view of things and decide to give up. But in a Sweet Chestnut state we do what we can to avoid giving up and look for a way out of our difficulties. If ill, we try different cures and therapies; if out of work we apply for jobs and overcome endless rejection; if alone, we make real efforts to meet people and make

> The experience of pain and distress formed a thick layer between what I was doing and the me beneath. It blocked the natural energy flow in part for years. Sweet Chestnut eased away the experience of pain and there being no way out. – Susan Rigg
>
> Sometimes people do not recover and die, but even death can be a very healing experience when the person resolves his emotional blockages and dies in real peace. True healing doesn't merely mean the recovery of physical health.
> – Nobuko Asanuma

friends. But despite our every effort no avenue opens to us and at last we face the awful fact that there is nothing more to be done. This is the point when we are most vulnerable: the dark night of the soul in anguish, when, in Bach's words, 'it seems there is nothing but destruction and annihilation left to face.' We don't choose despair; it is thrust upon us. At these moments Sweet Chestnut can be the gleam of unexpected light that leads us back to harbour.

the unexpected

Yesterday we took our children to school, went to work, had lunch with a friend, bought a newspaper, came home to our partner and our children, phoned our parents. We get up this morning expecting today to turn out much the same.

Suddenly something happens. Life twists away into something awful and strange. A parent dies, or a child or a neighbour. Or our company tells us not to come to work any more. Or the newspaper tells of war. Or our partner leaves us. We know as a rational fact that people lose their jobs and their lives and their peace and their loved ones every day. But knowing it in the mind is different from feeling it in the stomach. So that when something happens, and happens *to us*, it always finds us unprepared. It floods us, breaks the barriers, and stops us in our tracks. How to move forward? How to cope? The stock answer is to grieve and let go. But what if the shock stuns us so that we can't grieve properly? What if our grief is too wide to be crossed, so there seems to be no comforting harbour at the far side?

comfort yourself: star of bethlehem

A common French name for star of Bethlehem is *la dame d'onze heures*, a reference to the fact that the flowers open late in the morning when the sun is well up in the sky. The idea of an eleventh-hour plant reminds us that Star of Bethlehem can be an emergency remedy, something to be reached for at moments of crisis and trauma. Consequently it is a key ingredient in Rescue™ Remedy. But as the main flower against shock and its after-effects Star of Bethlehem is much more than a quick fix.

The effects of shock don't always appear at once and are not always obvious when they do. We may think that we have got over a trauma and are fully recovered but unresolved shock can remain buried deep in our hearts and will surface eventually. Philip Chancellor gives some examples in his *Illustrated Handbook*: a healthy woman sheltering on cellar steps in an air raid, and later developing arthritis as a result; another, also caught in an air raid, and a year later developing head pains, swollen glands and vision problems; a musician who traced a number of health problems back to an incident where she was accused of something she hadn't done. In all these cases Star of Bethlehem helped to get the minds and hearts of these people working again so they could accept what had happened and move on. (Chancellor goes on to suggest that Star of Bethlehem is worth considering whenever other essences have been ineffective, on the grounds that there might be some hidden shock at the root of the apparent problems. The Bach Centre teaches, and I agree, that we should only do this as a last resort. As a rule it is much better to select right remedies for what is clearly there and allow buried shock to come to the surface in its own time. This has the advantage of taking longer, allowing us time to learn about our emotions as they are revealed one by one.)

One kind of shock we will all face at some time is the loss of a loved one. The good and healing response to bereavement is to grieve, and society shows wisdom in allowing an interval between death and the funeral. The time of mourning is a retreat from normal life. We stop thinking about everyday concerns – sport, work, television – and instead have space to come to terms with our loss and understand what it means to us. And at the end of this time we bury or cremate the remains of the person we have lost – a symbolic end to the period of introspection after which we can begin to move on, changed and tempered by our experiences. Star of Bethlehem doesn't take grief away, nor should it. But it will help us get through the grieving process so that we don't become stuck in it, so that our loss doesn't override the normal process of bereavement and rebirth back into life. Like the star that led the wise men to the infant Jesus this flower is a remedy of hope and comfort, and a guide in the darkest night.

Without question my most notable success with the remedies occurred about five years ago. I attended an adventure weekend with our local youth club in the Lake District. It was wet and cold. One day I fell on a slippery bank and landed on my coccyx. At the time I experienced no pain, but several weeks later I became aware of a nagging ache. I ignored it, but it got worse over the next few months and it became difficult to sit comfortably; I felt as though I was sitting on a stone. Over the next year I tried homoeopathy, physiotherapy and osteopathy, all to no avail. One day I decided to take Star of Bethlehem for the original trauma of the fall. After four weeks the pain disappeared completely. – Maggie

this month in oxfordshire

This month in Oxfordshire – it is December – the weathermen say we have had the wettest end to a year since records began. Here in Wallingford flooding threatens only a few houses – further downstream people have been less fortunate – but the Thames is still the highest I have seen it in the ten years I have lived here.

Today the waters started to go down at last after a few days of little and light rain. Some of the overflow has drained away, leaving mud and dirt slopped into every hollow. The dark rain clouds have gone. Instead fog and mist and muggy grey blears the town. Every breath is full of dirty water, and the ground is saturated. Coming across the river bridge from Crowmarsh at about half past three in the afternoon, as the light began to fail, the clouds, the water, the mud and the gloom made everything dingy and colourless, even the Christmas decorations lit up over the shops. The streets and the people looked as though a slipshod cleaner had wiped a mop of grey water over them. Even the air was smeared, streaked and bespattered.

It would be good, I thought, to get a hose and connect it to a summer stream full of clean fresh spring water and wash down the town and the air and the people and leave them sparkling new again. For a moment I was caught up in how dull and tired it all looked. But my daughter had just finished her last day at school and was looking forward to getting home and to Santa Claus, and suddenly so was I.

love yourself: crab apple

Apples and apple blossom have long been associated with youth and rejuvenation. In Norse mythology the gods kept their youth by eating golden apples supplied to them by the goddess Iduna. The evil god Loki enticed Iduna away; the gods grew old and spring was delayed until she and the apples were restored. In Wales mourners used to lay apple blossom on corpses before burial to ensure the renewal of youth in the afterlife. The flower essence made from the white blossoms of *Malus pumila* does not claim to restore youth. But it does help us look at ourselves with a kinder and more childlike eye, so that we can accept the way we look and the things we feel.

In the classic Crab Apple state we feel ugly or unclean. The reason for this might be something we have done or something that we are or simply the way we look. Whichever the thing we pick on we feel that if we could only change this one thing and cleanse it from us then everything else would be fine. The one small spot preys on our minds and gets out of proportion so that we miss the heart of things. Even healthy physical functions like sex and eating are sometimes seen as 'dirty' and somehow improper.

By extension the Crab Apple state sometimes appears as a kind of fussy, house-proud over-concentration on unimportant external details, often to the exclusion of things that are more essential or more positive. We might endlessly dust and rearrange our books but never actually read one. Or we spend our time picking tiny weeds out of our front drive while our children fail at school for lack of support. Or we must vacuum the hall carpet again before going out even though doing so means arriving late for the party. As these examples suggest the Crab Apple attention to detail is often focused on dirt and contamination.

Crab Apple helps us to rise above trivial problems and get a truer perspective on life. We can judge better what is important and not get overly concerned about trifles. Once we have turned our attention away from unimportant things (the hall carpet) and things that we can do little about (the shape of our eyes) we can start to deal with the real business of life: developing ourselves and helping others. This is what Ian did, with the help of the practitioner who tells his story.

Ian's problem was his hair. It was falling out, and he was distraught. He came to see me on the advice of his GP. Amongst the remedies we chose two stood out. These were Rock-Water (his type remedy) and Crab Apple. I showed him how to make up a treatment bottle and because he was so concerned about his hair loss I suggested he add Crab Apple to his shampoo as well.

I didn't see Ian again until December, by which time he was completely bald. Even his eyebrows were gone. He had stuck religiously to his 'four drops four times a day' routine (no doubt due to his Rock-Water nature) and came to see if I could do another consultation. I thought he would want to talk about the hair loss again, the same as last time. I was wrong.

'You might not recognise me,' he said. 'I came in the summer because my hair was falling out. It's not my hair that's the problem, though – it's me!'

He said he felt his hair would start growing soon, but that didn't really bother him any more. His main intent was to discover what he could do to become a better person and so go forward positively in life.

In a negative Crab Apple state we equate progress with control of the one thing that obsesses us. In the positive state we lose our obsession and get a truer sense of what to notice and what to put aside. The world is clean and wholesome to us, from the clouds to the good honest dirt under our feet, and we embrace all of it. We love our bodies for what they are and enjoy being in our skin. Ian looked deeper into the mirror and saw beyond the surface. Crab Apple kicked off his journey.

I suffered from recurrent thrush. I took the medication and went on the diets but it always came back after a few weeks. I decided to take Crab Apple as I was feeling yuck about the condition, and it helped me remember the first time I suffered from it. I travelled across Asia during my early twenties and in some countries the men in the streets would grab me on the breasts and bottom. I felt disgusted and dirty, my body responded, and I had my first experience with thrush. To this day I still have not had the thrush return. I now know the wonder of Crab Apple. – Dianne Bradley

choose generosity: willow

Willow trees have a remarkable ability to grow roots. A branch stuck in the ground will turn into a new tree with little care and attention, so that even novice gardeners can create fences of living willow by planting fresh-cut poles. The Bible tells how the Jews hung their harps on willow trees during their exile in Babylon. Folklore adds that the weight of the harps caused the branches to droop and look forlorn, which is why the best-known type of willow, *Salix babylonica*, is commonly called the weeping willow. By extension all willows are associated with sorrow, including the type that makes the Willow remedy, *Salix vitellina*. Somebody who 'wears the willow' is mourning a lost love, and not necessarily one lost to death.

Like the trees the Willow state takes root with remarkable ease, often arising out of some other remedy state or characteristic: the injured self-regard of Chicory, for example, or the preoccupation with one's problems shown by Heather. Willow's unhappiness comes from too much negative regard being given to the good things in other people's lives. Negative Willow feels everyone else has something she doesn't – it could be money, looks, promotion, good hair – and so feels unhappy and hard done by and full of self-pity. She begrudges the good fortune of other people and sulks and complains. Life isn't fair to her in particular and everything is somebody else's fault. And if other people try to help her or cheer her up she is ungrateful. She takes the offered help as a right and is always ready to find fault for the things that have *not* been offered. She is the last to notice any improvement in her condition and the first to see where things are not as they should be.

We are responsible for our own unhappiness. And by the same token the cure for it lies in our own hands, not other people's. In a Willow state the answer is as simple as focusing on the things we *do* have so as to find our own reasons to be content. In his book *Powers of the Soul* Tom Meyer describes an exercise that he uses in his seminars to make this same point. He starts by asking people to write down twenty-five things they feel they need in order to be truly happy. Most people include things like winning the lottery, owning fast cars or private aeroplanes, big houses, beautiful partners. Then he asks them to write down the twenty-five things in their current lives that they are most happy to have. People's second columns typically list healthy children, loving partners, eyes, legs, hands, good health. Finally he asks his students to compare the two lists and answer a simple question: Would they give up the things on the second list in order to get the things on the first? And the answer, always, is 'no'. The positive things we have are always more important than the things we think we need. As Meyer puts it, 'happiness means taking pleasure in what you have.'

Positive Willow sees this and acts on it. But she goes further and rejoices in the good fortune of others. She is open and gives credit where it is due. She has no bitterness in her. She is an expression of love and generosity. She can laugh when things go wrong. The true willow is not weeping at all but full of life and regeneration. In winter, when all is dark and gloomy, the bare twigs of *Salix vitellina* turn a vivid orange-yellow and shine out in the countryside.

> The reality of life is that it's not easy. No one gets through unscathed or has an easy ride. When we accept this, life is a little easier because we don't feel so hard done by. – Alison Lock
>
> I spent a whole day composing an essay for a correspondence course and asked my husband to give me an opinion of my work. He showed me all the things I had done wrong. I was terribly resentful, thinking, I am obviously not cut out for this. I might just as well give up. After an hour of fuming I sipped a glass of water containing Willow and began to realise he was only trying to help and was actually right. I did need to rewrite it again with more thought. – Cynthia Prior

st christopher

St Christopher is the patron saint of travellers and load-bearers. According to legend his original name was Offero. He was a pagan – his father dedicated him to Apollo and another god called Machmet – who grew up famous for his great size, bravery and obstinacy. Proud of his strength, he left home to seek adventures and find service with the strongest and bravest master in the world, as only the greatest would be worthy of his service.

The first master he chose for himself was a powerful king. But he found that the king was frightened of the devil. So he left his human master and served the devil instead. For a time he wandered the world in the devil's company and was content to see how all bowed before him. But one day they came near a cross erected by the roadside. The devil grew pale and refused to pass by. Thus Offero realised there was another master stronger even than the devil. At once he put the devil behind him and sought a way to serve this greater master.

His wandering took him to a deep and dangerous river. There he found a hermit who helped travellers by pointing out safe ways to cross the torrent; without his help many would have been swept away and lost. The hermit heard Offero's tale and told him that the great master he sought was Christ, and that the way to serve him was to fast and pray and help others as he did. Offero accepted Christ as master and stayed with the hermit, taking his place after his death. But instead of merely showing people how to cross he used his great strength to battle the raging waters and carry travellers across on his back. This was safer for them, and the risk to himself he discounted: he had been given the body of a giant and it was his duty to use it to support others.

One day a tiny child came to the hut where Offero lived and asked to be shown the way across the river. Offero answered that he would carry him across.

'Can you bear my weight?' asked the child.

The giant Offero looked down and laughed and said that he could. Bending down, he grasped the child under his arms and pulled him up and set him on his shoulders. He was surprised at his great weight, which was more than a normal man's, but it wasn't more than he could manage.

They began to cross the stream. The further they went the heavier the child grew. After a time Offero staggered and almost fell.

'Set me down if I am too heavy,' said the child.

Offero refused. He staggered on a little further, the waters buffeting his legs, his knees trembling.

'Set me down and rest if you must,' said the child.

Again Offero refused. And at last, when he was on the point of collapse and the veins stood out on his arms and his back was cracking, they got to the far bank, and Offero gladly placed the child, dry, on the far side.

'Who are you that weigh as great as the world?' asked Offero.

'I am Christ, the creator and redeemer,' said the child. 'And you have borne the weight of the world upon your shoulders.'

Christ baptised Offero into his service and named him Christopher, a name which means 'Christ bearer'. He told Christopher to plant his staff in the ground, and by the next morning it had grown into a mighty tree that was a source of wonder throughout that country. But the miracle and Christopher's popularity angered the local heathen king. He had Christopher arrested and tortured and put to death. Christopher died without renouncing his faith, and was canonised by popular acclaim.

In 1969 the Catholic Church reviewed its calendars of saints and looked at the historical evidence for the existence and holiness of each one. When the commission charged with this duty came to Christopher they found that the evidence was very scanty. Somebody who might have been Christopher had died a martyr in the third century. The rest was conjecture. Unlike some other 'saints' who proved to be entirely legendary, Christopher was not suppressed entirely. But he was demoted and removed from the universal calendar of saints. No doubt if he were alive he would bear this indignity just as he bore so much else.

measure your strength: oak

When Bach wrote of 'the perseverance of the Oak which braved all tempests, offering shelter and support to the weaker things', he became part of a long tradition that associates oak with strength and resilience. Oak is endowed with magical properties, the tree of mighty gods like Thor, Jupiter and Zeus. Shipbuilders have long cherished the strength and durability of its timber and the way it resists storm and lightning strike alike (any tree beloved of the thunder gods must expect to be struck from time to time). Oak doors, floors, furniture and panelling all evoke solidity, strength and endurance, as well as a certain ponderous dignity. The oak is slow-growing and long-lived – the Cowthorpe Oak near Wetherby in Yorkshire is said to be over 1,600 years old – and in Britain it supports more forms of life, from lichen to insects to birds, than any other tree. It supports people too. Stories abound of people hiding from danger in its branches – Charles II is only the most famous – and even holding dinner parties inside the hollows of still-living trees.

The positive Oak state is one in which we feel strong and capable and able to bear great burdens without cracking. We never give up hope. We handle whatever life throws at us, and because we have strength enough and to spare we can help those around us to deal with their troubles as well. But at the same time we are aware of our needs. Like Christopher we know when we have done all we can, and find a safe place to set down our burden before our strength fails. This allows us to be measured in all things: steady and reliable when working, and calm and peaceful when it is time to rest.

Oak helps rebalance us when our natural strength leads us to struggle on beyond our limits. Perhaps through a sense of duty, perhaps through a lack of self-awareness, we deny ourselves rest and continue to work at the same relentless, steady pace, plodding on and on until eventually the heart of oak snaps. If we reach this point we can fall all at once into complete despair because when the oak does fail it breaks completely; it isn't uncommon for true Oak types to move suddenly into a Sweet Chestnut state after many years of faithful determination. With measured use of the remedy at the right time we hope never to reach this point.

We sometimes need to draw on the positive qualities of Oak while we are actually making it. Male and female flowers grow alongside each other on oak trees. The male flower forms a long droopy cluster that is easy to see and would quickly fill a remedy-making bowl. We don't use it. Instead we use the pinhead-sized female flower, which grows tucked behind the leaves out of sight. Finding a flower is a challenge in itself, and it can take a whole morning to cover the surface of just one bowl of water. One needs determination, thoroughness and a refusal to give in to an aching back and the heat of the sun.

> My first dose of Oak and I felt a huge weight had been lifted off my shoulders. – Theresa McInnes

know your power: elm

Positive Elm is like the mature tree: upright, tall and strong, stately and unshakeable, in legend a conductor of powerful magic. Elm is secure in herself. She knows her own strength and the path she wants to take. This usually turns towards the needs of others, because Elm is capable and responsible, able to deal with many demands and meet her own high expectations and the needs of others. But like the tree, which has been wiped out in parts of England due to the ravages of Dutch elm disease, Elm has a flaw, a weak spot that can undo her power. At times the sheer weight of her responsibilities appals her and shatters her confidence and strength. In the negative state she feels that nobody could be expected to deal with so many problems and duties. It seems beyond the strength of any human being. She feels exhausted and despondent, and her tasks, each one so easy in itself, add up to a burden that seems beyond her abilities. Her depression is all the greater because up to now she has been in love with her work. The thought that she can no longer cope with it is cruel indeed.

When we fall into this state, and it is the number of our responsibilities that causes our problem rather than over-enthusiasm or a lack of interest in what we are doing, then Elm is the correct flower to help us regain our positive certainty of success. Our reserves are limitless once we are in balance, and we will find the strength we need to recover. The negative Elm state is only ever a temporary condition. The sooner we use the remedy to reconnect with our reserves of self-belief the more temporary that condition can become. In this we are luckier than the tree, which never recovers from Dutch elm disease.

> I discovered Elm when I developed lower back pain and felt as though I'd seized up completely; this coincided with a time at work when I felt particularly stressed and unable to cope. I tried various analgesic rubs and anti-inflammatories and then I had a mental picture of a tree bent over in the wind and I used Elm. I don't know how long it took but I suddenly realised the pain had gone. – Theresa McInnes

dropping the balls

I was attending an evening class for parents who wanted to help their five- and six-year-old children enjoy reading and writing. One mother told us about her son. He had been slow to begin reading, and when he started school things got worse. His first teacher – made irritable by illness – held him up in front of the other children as an example of how *not* to read and how *not* to write. She was impatient when he stumbled over words, never praised him when he got things right, was always lying ready to pounce on the first mistake. Now he refused to read at all.

It sounds like an extreme case and a form of cruelty, but many of us learn at a much younger age that getting things wrong is bad. 'Naughty boy' and 'bad girl', the constant hymn of harassed parents, teaches us that making a mistake means more than *doing* something wrong – it means *being* wrong, *being* a failure. We become fearful of making mistakes and begin to base our sense of self-worth on our ability to succeed first time out. We avoid failure by only doing the things that we know we can do. And if we fail at something that we thought we could do... then better avoid doing it again. This can be a curiously comfortable position to adopt. If we assume that we are no good at something, assume that we are less talented, less able, less gifted, that absolves us of responsibility. We don't need to try if the result is a foregone failure. We can sit back and let the other guy take over.

This is no way to achieve success because in reality failure is part of the process of winning. During those times when we feel stuck or think we are getting worse our unconscious minds continue to re-evaluate and re-combine our experiences in preparation for the next leap forward. Every step along the path provides new information, even if at times we seem to be moving away from where we wanted to go. Failure, stagnation and lack of progress are part of our evolution, as long as we never give up, as long as we know that in the end we can expect to succeed.

In their book *Lessons from the Art of Juggling* Michael Gelb and Tony Buzan use the metaphor of juggling to explore how failure helps learning. Making mistakes in juggling means dropping the balls. But we can run all round the room in a panic and manage to catch the balls and still be bad jugglers. The secret of juggling is not *catching the balls* at all – it's throwing them so well that the hand can catch them without effort. In the early stages of juggling, say Gelb and Buzan, we learn better if we fail on purpose, and allow the balls to drop so as to concentrate on throwing right. In other words, we need to think about the process (the throw) more than the result (the catch).

Instead of fearing mistakes we need to embrace them, welcome them; even, at times, create them on purpose. Deliberately making mistakes is a way of breaking out of old patterns and finding new ones. Buzan once threw a ball too high by mistake so that it bounced off the floor instead of landing in his hand. But as it rose and fell again he caught it in rhythm and his juggling continued uninterrupted. The 'mistake' became part of his act. So why not deliberately drop the balls, deliberately invite failure, deliberately fracture a successful pattern from time to time to see what new information it provides and what new things there are to be learned? If we don't try we'll never know. And if we do try, on purpose, to fail, we can pick a time and place where our failure will not do real damage. Given the right teacher the five-year-old boy could have been inspired by the trips and mispronunciations in the texts he was reading. They could all have been an invitation to notice something and explore further.

expect success: larch

We need Larch when we lose confidence in our ability to do things well. Convinced that our talents are not great enough to win through, we refuse to try and accept defeat before it happens. We compare ourselves with others and find ourselves wanting. We avoid opportunities and responsibilities. We believe we lack the talent to do as well as other people and our belief excuses us from even trying. Caught between despair and false modesty we live lives lacking in adventure and risk and waste our potential for good and for growth in a self-effacing mediocrity.

'Let us not fear to plunge into life,' said Bach. 'We are here to gain experience and knowledge, and we shall learn but little unless we face realities and seek to our utmost.' Larch incarnates those qualities of confidence and self-belief that allow us to follow this advice. Larch plunges up to her neck in life and knows that whatever happens will be for the best. As long as she lives fully and takes her chances when they come she can accept failure and success with equanimity. Mistakes are just part of her progress. She takes pleasure in them, invites them, and plays with life.

The larch tree is the only coniferous tree to lose its leaves in winter. Its branches droop before turning up at the end, giving the tree as a whole the look of somebody giving a helpless shrug and a silent question, 'What can *I* do?' The answer of the Larch flower is: whatever you want. Larch tells us we are as good as everyone else. We will succeed in our own time and way.

A particularly vivid dream occurred after taking a combination that included Larch. I was flying and suddenly found myself in America, hovering above the Sandia Mountains in New Mexico. There was a tremendous sense of peace and well-being, it felt warm and safe. I said, 'Anything is possible – I can do anything,' and really believed it. Apart from being extremely pleasant it turned out to be a most helpful and inspiring dream. In fact it changed my life. – Lynne Crescenzo

Within a few weeks of taking Larch an extraordinary thing happened. I decided to learn to swim. Several years before I had attempted to learn and given it up as hopeless, but this time I knew I could master it. And I did. It's an achievement I take great pleasure in relating to all and sundry. – Jill Woods

value your efforts: pine

A sense of natural justice is a source of light and a power for good. It lets us weigh and reflect on our experiences so we can learn from them and make things better. But in a negative Pine state justice gives way to judgement, and so to condemnation – and it is all directed against ourselves.

Guilt is like black pigment added to a pot of coloured paint, in that it doesn't take much to make dark and forbidding what was bright and clear. From a position where we blame ourselves for one error the darkness spreads until we see everything as our fault. 'Sorry' is forever on our lips, even when somebody else is to blame, and it remains there when things go right. However well we may have done we see the imperfections rather than the achievement and condemn ourselves for not having done better still.

Of all negative emotions guilt is one of the most destructive. It corrodes our sense of self-worth. It stops us from taking pleasure ('I don't deserve this pleasure') and tells us that we are fundamentally worthless and to blame ('I deserve all the pain I get'). It leads us to take on the burden of other people's mistakes, which denies us the joy we deserve and denies them the chance to take responsibility for their actions. And it stops progress. Instead of accepting the inevitability and desirability of failure and allowing it to take us forward we spend our energies spiralling around events that would be better dealt with or forgotten.

With the help of the Pine essence we can begin to lighten the picture again. In a positive state we have a clearer and truer picture of where our responsibility lies and where it finishes. If we have done wrong we can acknowledge the fact without assuming that one bad action makes us guilty for ever. We can try to put a wrong right and if this is not possible we can seek forgiveness and, just as important, forgive ourselves. If other people have done wrong we can help them share the burden but we still understand and make clear that it is their burden and not ours. We will see that true kindness towards others means allowing them to take responsibility for their mistakes and learn from them, just as we take responsibility for and learn from our own.

7 ❀ steps along the path

who we are

Nora Weeks was the first of many writers to recommend that we think about the qualities we admire in other people as a way of pinpointing areas we need to work on. So if our hero were some energetic and enthusiastic politician who was good with words, persuasive and a campaigner for justice, and *if we really were lacking in energy and enthusiasm*, then we could think about Hornbeam or Larch or Wild Rose to see if they represent positives that we need to develop. Thinking about changing our personality in this way – in other words, developing the qualities we lack – has always been part of selecting essences. But there are two important limits to this approach:

❀ *First*, the second 'if' (*if we really were lacking in energy and enthusiasm*) is crucial. Wild Rose and Hornbeam won't help us if we are already pumped full of enthusiasm and only want more energy so as to continue burning the candle at both ends. We must beware of backing our more out-of-balance aspirations. Humility and a willingness to be honest about our existing faults are essential prerequisites for using the essences wisely.

❀ *Second*, we must be realistic about who we can be. Our task on earth is not to become somebody completely different. Instead it is to be ourselves so that we can learn from our lives. We may admire the politician's qualities and want to develop similar qualities in ourselves, but that doesn't mean forgetting who we are and trying to take on her personality.

We all know how our environment affects the way we express ourselves. A good environment allows us to develop what we have to
great heights. A bad one can deform us until we appear utterly different from who we are. But whether expressed or deformed, who we are
remains the unchanging key. The idea that everybody can or should
develop in the same way — six-packs, white teeth, identical positive-
thinking and extrovert minds — is fundamentally flawed. Our task is
not to become somebody different. Rather it is to learn about and
accept who we are. For we don't just have 'a personality'. In Bach's
words, we have 'a *glorious* personality, a *wonderful* individuality' (my
emphasis). Once we peel away all the negative traits and habits that we
think make up our personality we will discover that our true personality is more amazing than we ever suspected. And the reason for this
is that the personality, the real on-course personality, is an expression
of the soul, the divine, the spirit, the pure man.

The need to uncover this glorious and unique personality
explains why the path to genuine growth has nothing to do with the
one-step-to-greatness-all-together-now delusions of the self-help
video guru. Genuine growth always involves greater knowledge of
our individual selves (learning how we really feel, learning who we
really are). This is a personal path that each of us treads in our
hearts. 'I see my relationship with the remedies as part of a continuing
exploration,' says Ian McPherson, a hypnotherapist who has been
using the system for about seven years. 'As old issues are resolved new
ones arise, and over the years I have greatly increased my awareness of
my own character and personal processes, confident in the knowledge
that the remedies support me in doing this.' We are probably not sure
who we are when we start but we get a clearer picture as the remedies
help us see ourselves more clearly. 'Working with the remedies means
setting out on an intensive process of self-discovery,' says Miki
Hayashi, another practitioner who uses the essences in her work.
'Often the flower we most need is the one whose soul quality we

are least able to relate to. We tend to be blind to our own character traits.'

Step by step, aware of every step: this is the way out of the blindness and towards the heart of who we are.

type remedies

The thirty-eight essences all express a movement from negative to positive. Each of them relates to our passing moods, helping us find out how we feel and express our most positive qualities. And some of them – the type remedies – go deeper. They relate to essential personality characteristics. In the language of the flowers they define who we are.

Take Agrimony as an example. All of us fall into a negative Agrimony state from time to time (we joke about the end of a relationship to hide the pain), just as we sometimes express the positive aspects (we are open about our loss while retaining our sense of humour). But some of us will have a tendency to display these negative and positive states more often, and for us Agrimony may be our type remedy. To see this is true, think now of a few Agrimony people you have known or read about or seen on television. The chances are you can think of several people who incarnate the classic Agrimony qualities – those smiling, sociable people, the light-hearted jokers, the party-goers. It's probable too that you will find it easier to think of negative Agrimony types than of positive ones, simply because the negative characteristics stick out more. (If you can't think of any, here are some suggestions, in no particular order, and of course you can disagree if you knew them personally! – the American film icon Marilyn Monroe, the British comedians Frankie Howerd and Kenneth Williams, and the ex-President of Russia, Boris Yeltsin.)

Even the most clear and obvious Agrimony person will need other essences from time to time. Marilyn Monroe might have benefited from Walnut if the attention of the fans got too much for her. Boris Yeltsin might have needed Impatiens if he felt that reforms weren't going fast enough – and would certainly go faster if only people would leave it to him! But the need for these essences will come and go and often be associated with specific events or moments in life: a failed audition, a meeting with an over-cautious economist. The type remedy, in this case Agrimony, will be a recurrent thread in the person's life. And it will often precipitate rather than react to events. Perhaps Monroe feels under particular pressure from her fans because she always seemed so happy to see them in the past.

A clear explanation of the importance of type remedies appeared in the September 1970 issue of the Bach Centre Newsletter. Parts of it are quoted from Bach's writings, other parts are Nora Weeks's recollection of what he told her about type remedies.

We come to earth with a personality of our own, and our real work is to develop, improve, and as near as possible, perfect that personality; and for this work throughout life, our own remedy, the one relating to our own personality, will be needed to help us. For example, take a Vervain personality, his life's work is to modify and soften his intensity of purpose. That will be his life's work all the time. But at times he may come under the influence of others and forget his life's work, he may worry, become restless, qualities which the Vervain personality should never know, yet he may need the remedy Agrimony. Or he may find doubt creep into his mind, nothing more foreign to his personality, then he will need Gentian. Most of us at some time or other become open to outside influence, and it is then that we need the remedy which protects us against that particular danger, but always we need help from our personality or type remedy, the one which will strengthen our determination to learn the particular lesson we have come to earth to learn.

As this passage says, the type remedy indicates the main fault we are here to work on. This is shown by the number of times problems in our lives turn out to be something to do with our type remedy. And it is shown too by the way we will often react in our type way to whatever provocation life throws at us. Faced with a boring party, a job to do or a troublesome child the Agrimony person will smile and make a joke, the Impatiens person will try to speed things up and cut corners, the Oak person will plod through without losing her temper or getting too excited. Those watching will look at each other and say, 'Typical'.

bach's type remedy

I don't know what Bach's type remedy was and I don't think it truly matters. So why ask the question? The answer is that I have heard various theories put forward, and even if none of them is conclusive that doesn't mean they have nothing to teach.

Some people have suggested Impatiens. Indications would include Bach's hurry to move away from the past (he destroyed his old notes every time his work advanced), his keenness to publish his findings at every stage and as soon as possible, and his quickness to break the rules of the General Medical Council if he felt they got in his way. 'There were times when he was inclined to become impatient,' writes Philip Chancellor,

> when others were not as quick as he was, and were slow to follow his line of thought. When this occurred, he had an immediate physical reaction, and a red and very irritating rash would suddenly appear. He would say: 'You see, my being irritable with you hurts me more than it hurts you!' A dose of Impatiens would restore his good humour, and within a short time the rash would disappear.

Cerato is another suggestion, although its supporters stress that Bach must have been a positive Cerato person and would not have needed to take the flower very often. Evidence for Cerato includes the fine and growing intuitive sense that led him to discover the true healing essences, his independence of thought, his ability to follow his heart despite what the world thought, and the fact that he never seems to have asked for advice but always strove to listen to his inner voice.

Chancellor reads these same characteristics in a slightly different way, and in doing so demonstrates how the positive aspects of different essences can appear to be very close to each other:

> Dr Bach himself was a good example of the Walnut type. He forsook all of his old ideas of healing to find a better way to cure people. He did this in spite of ridicule, lack of encouragement, and advice to the contrary, proffered by his old colleagues. He persevered even against the strong influence of his own training and background in medicine.

According to Chancellor, then, Bach was a positive Walnut most of the time. Weeks tells how Bach's sensitivity grew to such an extent that 'he was aware of the disease or complaint of the next patient who was to visit him [and] would contract the symptoms of the disease himself.' This would be an indication that he did need Walnut occasionally to help him resist these outside influences.

Other people think of Bach as Vervain: look at his wholehearted commitment to his beliefs and his efforts to communicate them to his patients and to the wider world through his books and lectures. Or he is an Oak, struggling on through his illness in 1917 and enduring great suffering at the end of his life when finding the last nineteen essences.

It's always much harder to spot somebody's type remedy when they are generally in balance. The difficulty that people have had defining Bach's type remedy perhaps indicates that he was more or less in balance most of the time, at least after he left London and began his life's work. This is only what we would expect of somebody who had successfully found his path in life. All we can say with any certainty is that Bach suffered all the remedy states at one time or another. We can say this with certainty because the same observation is true of all human beings who live beyond babyhood.

peeling the onion

If it's hard trying to make up our minds about somebody else's type remedy that doesn't mean we won't have as much trouble identifying our own. Layers of negative emotion can build up over the years, sometimes over a whole lifetime, and years of dissembling and subterfuge and posturing can make us believe we are different from who we really are. Sometimes we are led away by our own desires and fears, sometimes we adopt different behaviour so as to fit in with others. In the case of Jackie Lowy, a counsellor and former nurse, there was a mixture of both. 'I have never followed my own way for fear of being alone,' she says. 'I feared not having friends so I adapted my behaviour to suit them. After many years of doing this I lost who I really was.'

Even when our personality still shines out it may be warped by some emotional state or trauma that took root in the past and was never resolved. Like grit in an oyster this too can provoke the build-up of layers of imbalance. We may need to find and deal with this forgotten event before we can successfully express our true selves.

John Ramsell was the first to call the process of dealing with these layers 'peeling the onion', and the name has stuck. Peeling the onion means selecting flowers for whatever is clearly there now – today's emotions, today's issues, the outside of the onion – and allowing the essences to deal with these so as to reveal whatever is underneath. This reverses the process that led to the warping or concealment of our true selves. 'The remedies are my way of dis-covering myself,' says Lowy, while another essence user called Una found that past traumatic events came back to the surface in reverse order: 'As each emotion or event surfaced I used the remedies to help deal with them.' Peeling the onion is a process of self-discovery, an essential part of finding out how we feel, why we feel and who we are.

We never know what will be at the heart of our onion until we unpeel it. At its most dramatic we may discover some inner demon that we need to confront and conquer. David Whyte reads the sixth-century epic *Beowulf* as a parable for this kind of process: the warrior hero fights and kills the monster Grendel only to have Grendel's mother appear. (In more modern times the makers of films like *Godzilla* and *Aliens* have borrowed the same plot.) Facing and destroying one monster only provokes and uncovers a deeper and more dangerous monster, just as dealing with one out-of-balance emotion can uncover a second and more serious underlying imbalance. In Whyte's neat phrase, 'it is not the thing you fear that you must deal with, it is the mother of the thing you fear.'

Whatever we expect or hope or fear to find we must trust what is always true, that the remedies will only teach us when we are ready to learn. If the readjustment of an emotion uncovers the mother of fear that means we are ready to meet it and, like Beowulf, wrestle with it. The process of slow unpeeling gives us the time we need to learn about our feelings and prepare to meet them. The end is always positive. 'I have learned to become a friend to myself, instead of an enemy,' says Anna Richardson, who started using the essences in 1992. 'I have learned about the qualities of my character and how destructive they are when they are used negatively and how constructive they can be when used positively. I now seek the good within everyone, myself included, instead of mostly the bad.'

fun and fulfilment

This is all very earnest and may even seem scary. It shouldn't. If the journey crosses dark places it is always towards the light, and people stretch their legs every day for the sheer pleasure of it. As one remedy taker says, 'It isn't always easy to walk confidently along our path, but the remedies make the journey a little more fun.'

The rewards and joy of walking start anew with every step. Above all there is the feeling of *rightness*, the sense that we are going in directions we most need to go. 'My life has changed so much since my introduction to the remedies,' says Tracey Deacon. 'I now feel I am once again following the correct path for me. I have developed so much and feel a much more wholesome and complete individual with so much to give to others.'

Step by step, aware of every step: this is the way.

last and first men

In 1930 Olaf Stapledon, a Liverpudlian star-gazer and adult education teacher with degrees in philosophy and history, published a fictional book about the future of the human race. He called it *Last and First Men*.

Last and First Men is an unusual work, light-years from most people's idea of science fiction. The narrator is a historian, unimaginably far in the future, and the book is his scholarly account of humanity's development. The story starts more or less in our present, but in the eyes of this future historian we in the twenty-first century are not 'true' humans at all. We are just the first step on an evolutionary path, the First Men, only remarkable for a short-sighted technological obsession that exhausted our fuel reserves in the blink of an eye.

According to the historian, the spiritual high point of our species came long after our materialistic civilisation collapsed and we entered an age of decay and degeneracy. During this darkness, in about AD

100,000, a new sub-species flourished briefly in Patagonia. Patagonian men and women lived to seventy years of age, but their fire and spirit and flexibility had drained by the time they were fifteen. Its brevity made youth seem all the more precious, so much so that a religion formed around the cult of a legendary child, an eternal adolescent, God-the-favourite-child rather than God-the-father. This legend was based on a real and unusually vigorous Patagonian who once found himself trapped in a blizzard on a high mountain and sinking into a snowdrift − a literal peak experience. At first he fought to get free, raging at the thought of dying, but then he began to see himself from outside as if he were an actor in a play. He saw that whether he got free or died the play itself would be the better for his having lived and struggled in that moment. The game transcended the individual experiences of the players. Drawing strength from the sense of rightness and spiritual freedom that this insight gave him, he fought free and was able to bring news of his revelation to others. 'While I was a boy, I said, "Grow more alive",' he told them, 'but in those days I never guessed that there was an aliveness far intenser than youth's flicker, a kind of still incandescence.' (We are reminded of Abraham Maslow's later writings on peak and plateau experiences.)

In time the First Men fell away utterly and over millions of years the titanic Second Men flourished and died. Then came the Third Men, feline creatures with highly developed senses, an acute and practical intelligence, and a great interest in and love for all forms of life and nature. The Third Men built many great and wonderful civilisations, but the historian concentrates on one in particular, a culture based on music. Blessed with wonderful hearing, music had a spiritual appeal for the Third Men that we with our blunter senses can't begin to understand. Through music they achieved direct and mystical communion with each other. One especially gifted individual founded a church of music, which preached that the living soul of the universe was a kind of symphony and that each individual soul had its melody. Once sung, that melody lived for ever; from the view-point of a god nothing was ever lost. The way to immortality was to awaken our individual soul and to sing out as clearly and naturally as possible.

We pass over the Fourth Men, massive brains created artificially by the Third Men, but incapable of understanding life because they were trapped in their artificial environments. Their finest moment came when they understood their own limitations and created the Fifth Men.

The Fifth Men could live up to 3,000 years and enjoyed telepathic communication with each other. Thanks to their long lifetime and excellent health, and to a well-organised society that brought universal material wealth, they were able to spend most of their time on artistic and spiritual and philosophical concerns. Indeed, to them the three pursuits were one and the same, for they saw the whole universe as an infinitely complex work of art, continually developing in space and time. No human being could appreciate the completeness of the universe, but created art allowed parts of it to be understood and in part appreciated.

Over the tens of millions of years of their zenith the Fifth Men gained great insight into the macroscopic shifts of art and knowledge. They noticed how culture continually developed and changed, but not in a linear way. Development was a spiral. An area of study would be plumbed to its absolute depths and when there seemed nothing more to find the best minds would move on to mine a new and more promising field. This process would continue from age to age as old and exhausted interests were abandoned for the sake of new workings. But there always came a time when attention would turn again to the first worked-out area. And always it was found that new questions – millions of undiscovered and unexplored caverns – appeared, as if by magic. Facts discovered in other areas were found to be unexpectedly relevant and had to be accounted for. Discoveries in one science revolutionised understanding in another and always the old understanding had to be rebuilt and reshaped. Every reworking found new and more beautiful approximations to the truth, and no word was ever the last word on anything. (We are reminded of Thomas Kuhn's later model of scientific discovery.)

Last and First Men goes on to tell of many more thousands of millions of years of history. Humanity abandons earth when the moon crashes into it, and moves first to Venus and then further out to Neptune when the sun expands and swallows the inner planets. The Last Men are the eighteenth species to carry human genes. And the last and greatest view of the universe that the Last Men have, just before the sun swells further and wipes them out for good, is again a musical metaphor. 'Man himself, at the very least, is music,' says Stapledon's historian, 'a brave theme that makes music also of its vast accompaniment, its matrix of storms and stars.'

lessons of the labyrinth

Let's highlight three of the main themes in Stapledon's book.

- ✻ *First*, the view of life as a wonderful and profoundly serious game that has intrinsic value.
- ✻ *Second*, the idea of the universe as an evolving work of art that needs the music of life and spirit if it is to reach its highest possible state.
- ✻ *Third and last*, the rejection of simple linear development and the wisdom of the spiral, an endless circle that re-sees, revisits, recreates and rebuilds old knowledge.

We can gather these ideas together in the image of the labyrinth. The labyrinth is an ancient symbol for growth and life, and a symbol too of initiation and full entry into the human condition. Seen from the outside the pattern is clear and understandable, and stands for completion and wholeness: the labyrinth is among the earliest forms of art. But to play the game we have to get inside it and allow ourselves to be a-mazed by its apparently random twists and turns. The voyage through the labyrinth symbolises our journey through life, full of dead-ends and mistakes that oblige us to go back over our steps and find new ways through. Every division in the path demands a decision and a change of direction, and often we get lost. We may feel that taking a new turning is the start of a new path, and indeed to us it is: the path always starts anew, there in front of our feet. But no matter what turning we take it is still the same labyrinth, our own, that we walk.

The wonder of a labyrinth lies in the time and space it occupies. As we proceed we cover more ground than we ever could if we walked in a straight line. The longer the labyrinth, the more times we double back on ourselves; the longer the journey the richer the life. If we tread every inch and can stay focused on every step we will have lived to the utmost. And at the centre – if we ever reach it – we hope to find self-knowledge and fulfilment. The centre of anything is the most sacred point and our goal – as we could see if we could stand above the maze and see the whole pattern – is to find our own centre, a centre for our lives, and so find or forge a meaning. And whether we reach that end or not, nobody who enters the labyrinth ever emerges unchanged.

The labyrinth has an especially resonant message for modern humanity, as Jacques Attali points out in his book *Chemins de sagesse*. Since the birth of the Industrial Revolution we have tried to speed things up, walk in straight lines, avoid detours and backtracks. We try to do things faster and faster so as to save more and more time. We look forward always: get this out of the way, then that, then the next thing. But to what end? For in our frenzied activity we forget that the real trick of time is not to save it but to spend it: stargazing, dancing, laughing, singing, talking with our children, reading, thinking, meditating, sitting quietly, listening to the world. Many of the things that waste time are actually the point of living. As Attali says, don't we all try to go as slowly as possible from birth to death? We should welcome every detour and change of direction that slows us down and lets us spend more of our precious time.

ruts

A rut is a groove in the ground into which the wheels fall. It too is a kind of labyrinth, but a closed one with no alternative paths, no exits and no centre. We rock back and forth in it like the pendulum of a clock, and our motion only makes the rut deeper. It soothes us, until our sleepiness takes away the will we would need to steer our way out. Cradled in a rut we swing from place to place, from meal to meal, from bedtime to bedtime, from Monday to Monday, and between tick and tock a year goes and we are still in motion back where we started.

Ruts happen when we allow habit and boredom to flourish and forget to give love and attention to what we are doing. This is what Edward Bach says:

The antidote for boredom is to take an active and lively interest in all around us, to study life throughout the whole day, to learn and learn and learn from our fellow-men and from the occurrences in life the truth that lies behind all things, to lose ourselves in the art of gaining knowledge and experience, and to watch for opportunities when we may use such to the advantage of a fellow-traveller. Thus every moment of our work and play will bring with it a zeal for learning, a desire to experience real things, real adventures and deeds worth while, and as we develop this faculty we shall find that we are regaining the power of obtaining joy from the smallest incidents, and occurrences we have previously regarded as commonplace and of dull monotony will become the opportunity for research and adventure. It is in the simple things of life – the simple things because they are nearer the great truth – that real pleasure is to be found.

A practitioner and teacher based in London, Caroline Hedicker sees the rut in action when her clients reach the point of making a change. 'On the verge of letting go of something we feel we want to hang on to it,' she says. 'Our worries, troubles, problems, traumas are like old friends. Letting go of them may involve a change, maybe a change we don't feel quite ready for or secure enough to face. So we cling to the dead wood for all we are worth rather than putting that energy into new growth.' A tick, we teeter on the upper edge and are almost free, a tock, we fall back.

In contrast, the kind of awareness Bach recommends brings out the uniqueness of each moment so that we uncover the hidden exits and discover new ways through. Our natural curiosity awakes and we make changes as naturally as we breathe. Change becomes an old friend, something to be welcomed and expected every day in the same way we welcome and expect a favourite TV programme and a drink before bedtime. Each change follows the spiral and takes us back to new old paths armed with greater knowledge. We can even welcome those changes that cause most fear, those that see us switching careers and outgrowing constrictive relationships. 'My partner of ten years and I have separated,' says Tracey Deacon. 'I am now living on my own, and I can't remember ever having been so contented.' Clean cuts like this are positive when they are the next natural step and help us and the people we love grow, as was the case with Tracey and her ex-partner. 'We are still best friends and we still have a deep respect for each other. We have both been able to flourish in our own lives now – a change for the better that would probably never have happened if I had not found the remedies.' The trick is to judge when freedom

demands we make a break and when it only asks for the simple pay-
ing of more and better attention. Even after years of neglect many
relationships flourish when we regain the power of taking joy from
small instances.

Step by step, aware of every step: this is the way to turn out of the
rut and back into the labyrinth.

alexander the great

Alexander the Great inherited the throne of Macedonia when his
father died. At once he started a war against the Persians in revenge for
their invasion of Greece a century and a half before. Taking his war to
the east he came to the kingdom of Gordium. Here the priests showed
him the magical and wonderfully complex knot with which the
ancient king Gordius had bound his chariot to its yoke. They told him
that whoever could untie the knot would have the right to rule over
the whole of the East. They expected him to try to understand how
the knot worked, as everyone else had in the past. But Alexander simply pulled his sword out and cut the rope and the knot to pieces.
'Cutting the Gordian knot' is now a stock phrase for resolving a sticky
problem by force or for avoiding it altogether.

Alexander's was a peculiarly modern approach. The knot is a
form of labyrinth, an invitation to knowledge and wisdom. The sword
stroke is a straight line – linear development, a literal short cut from
A to B. Many find it attractive because of its apparent simplicity. True,
it is minimalist, and it is quick, but do we want to live minimalist lives
and get those lives over with as quickly as we can? Alexander's
approach is simplistic rather than simple because it sacrifices value.
Life offers us a different kind of simplicity, one that has much more to
do with the labyrinth and the steady unpicking of the knot.

'Like many people I was looking for the perfect life just around
the corner,' says Hilary Leigh, who trained as a practitioner in 1996.

The Alexandrine approach to enlightenment is just that: turn a corner and we're there, right at the heart. It's a fantasy, like those films in which a writer taps away at a keyboard, finishing her book in one draft, typing from page 1 to 200 with a neat 'The End' added at the bottom. Real writing, like life, is full of reverses and changes of mind. I spent several weeks mixing up the topics in this book and trying to arrange them like a maze. It was a nice idea that resulted in logical spaghetti. So I spent another fortnight undoing what I had done. This wasn't wasted time. It was part of the path I had to walk to write *Bloom*. My doubling back, one step at a time, meant I was further on. I knew more about *Bloom* and about what it could and couldn't be. We find this pattern in every walk of life. So when Hilary Leigh began to take the remedies she didn't find a sudden utopia around the corner, but the start of a path with more corners to turn. 'I started taking each day as it comes,' she says. 'I started treating life as the journey it is, to be lived each day to the full regardless of fear and disappointment. Events come into one's life at the right time. I now accept what is and find that position easier to build on. Those years I thought wasted were in fact a lesson.'

According to chaos theory the most complex systems form around the simplest of rules. A seed can only contain so much coded information; by teasing out the rules scientists can program computers to 'grow' perfect leaves on a screen. All these programs do is apply the same simple rules over and over. The leaf is a complex miracle, as is the labyrinth, but it is created step by step and with a limited number of directions. True natural simplicity – a minimum of necessary rules, small steps repeated – leads to richness and complexity.

We are our own labyrinth and our own evolution. To explore our individuality and discover our potential we need to walk every inch of who we are and use the opportunity of a lifetime to grow. All of us have it in us to reach the stars and express our soul's music and join with the universe, but we must start from where we are and be prepared to develop slowly and take every step on our path even if it does not go immediately where we think it needs to. 'In general,' says Aileen Falconer, who has been using the remedies for ten years, 'we don't go from stumbling in the darkness to running unhindered in full light in one leap. Rather we gradually remove obstacles from our path and a glimmer of light begins to shine. We start to walk without falling so often, the light increases and finally we can move freely with full vision. The process of removing the obstacles, of finding the light, of learning how to walk is just as valuable as the final outcome.'

Alexander the Great remains a hero to many, especially those of a forceful and authoritarian mind. His short life was full of sword cuts; his empire unravelled as soon as he had gone.

Life is like climbing a mountain. There are hard ways as well as easy ways, and sunny days as well as windy or rainy days. If we decide to climb a mountain we first prepare clothes to keep warm and food so as not to starve. Nobody tries to climb without those preparations.

Some people ask if taking remedies means we escape from our problems to an easier way, indulge ourselves, depend on remedies and not face our issues properly. When I am asked that question, I often talk about the mountain. Even if we get enough support from our warm clothes and food it is still our individual responsibility to keep climbing.

Using Bach remedies is one way of wisdom for human beings. While we are climbing we cannot see where the tops of the mountains are. But the higher we climb the clearer we will see the peaks.

— Yurina Shiraishi, Bach practitioner, Tokyo

vii ❊ give freedom, get freedom

The love of liberty is the love of others; the love of power is the love of ourselves.
– William Hazlitt, nineteenth-century essayist and critic

five kinds of freedom

In an address given at Southport in February 1931 Edward Bach outlined his beliefs about individual freedom and the ills of modern life. He identified greed as the chief disease of Western civilisation. He included all the normal kinds of greed that one might expect – desire for wealth, for power and position, for comfort and material possessions – but one kind of greed he condemned as especially dangerous because of its spiritual effects. This was the desire to possess another person.

Possessing other people means influencing or controlling the actions of others to such an extent that we take away part or all of their freedom. Greed of this kind is so endemic to our way of life that we have almost made it into a virtue. Advertising executives, politicians and leaders of all kinds are valued precisely *because* they are able to possess, control and influence. Yet Bach was right – this is a peculiarly ruinous form of greed – and the reason is that the sword of possession cuts both ways at once.

❊ *First*, it stops other people from following their path in life and from developing their full potential in their own way. We might wonder how many Mozarts we have lost thanks to the well-meaning interference of others.

🌼 *Second*, possessing and controlling others corrupts the possessor and deforms the controller. Being obeyed is intoxicating, and commanders are enslaved by their addiction as much as drug addicts are by theirs.

The sword of letting go is also double-edged, for in giving liberty to others we liberate ourselves. And liberation is full of youth and vigour, as intoxicating as and more wholesome than any addiction. As one fifty-year-old remedy user pointed out, 'There is a wonderful sense of freedom in directing our own lives and letting others direct theirs – a freedom I haven't experienced since I was a teenager with the world at my feet.'

The five essences in Bach's seventh group all relate to this kind of freedom.

🌼 **Chicory** gives affection and help with no thought of return, and is quick to give loved ones room to grow even if that means they grow away from her.

🌼 **Vervain** is strong in her convictions but still able to question them. She will seek to persuade others and inspire them but can set rational limits to her idealism and effort.

🌼 **Beech** sees the good in other people's ways of life even where these differ from or contradict her own. She is quick to value and slow to condemn, and a voice for mutual tolerance.

🌼 **Vine** is a wonderful guide for those who are lost, but she always knows when to stand back and allow mistakes to be made if that is the best way for others to learn.

🌼 **Rock Water** is content to develop slowly, never seeking martyrdom, and knows that the example of her way of life will not necessarily be of use to other people.

Bach's heading for this group was 'over-care for the welfare of others', and the essences in it help us not to care too much about what other people do. Each quality is quick to assist when there is real need but slow to assume that she knows best. None of them will hurt others, all work gently and with due respect for difference, and if help is refused they will step back and wait rather than impose a solution.

love and let go: chicory

Chicory helps us when our need to be loved perverts our love for others so that we become greedy for love and attention. We love but we demand something back, such as duty, affection, loyalty and recognition. In order to be wanted we offer help in an insistent way and make it hard for people to refuse; if they *do* refuse we call it ingratitude. We feel that the people we love should be glad of our care and should show their gratitude by spending time with us and making us the centre of attention. We may slide into self-pity and become injured martyrs. How could they treat us so badly after all we have done? We may even become manipulative, exaggerating our suffering (though we might not be aware of it as exaggeration) so as to gain sympathy and put our loved ones in a more difficult position.

At this extreme negative Chicory is blind to the real needs of others and sees only from her own perspective. This led Philip Chancellor to refer to Chicory people as 'the vampires of humanity'; others have followed his example and demonised the Chicory person into a monster. Yet according to Bach the negative Chicory state is all too human, which is why real love is so hard for us to achieve.

What we call 'love' is a combination of greed and hate, that is, desire for more and fearing to lose. Therefore what we call 'love' must be ignorance. Real love must be infinitely above our ordinary comprehension, something tremendous, the utter forgetfulness of self, the losing of the individuality in the Unity, the absorption of the personality in the Whole.

Chicory encourages the blossoming of this more divine form of love that is 'the very opposite of self'. Positive Chicory has no thought of return or reward. She offers love unconditionally, and knows too how to stand back and allow other people to learn unhindered from their lives and mistakes. She never interferes or manipulates and her first thought is to give others their freedom and take joy in their decisions and growth. Positive Chicory qualities are among the highest. Selfless love is a Christ-like quality, and with the help of this flower all of us can find it within us.

Negative Chicory states happen to male and female, old and young: the schoolboy who threatens to be ill if he can't stay at home is in a negative Chicory state as much as the father who sulks if his son doesn't support the same football team. Nevertheless we often imagine the archetypal Chicory as a mother figure, perhaps because in most cultures we associate mother-hood (rather than fatherhood) with unconditional giving and selfless, out-ward-looking love. When love turns selfish in a mother it seems especially surprising and noteworthy. Maybe we expect less of men....

In some parts of Germany *Chichorium intybus* is known as 'watcher of the road' after a young girl who waited by a roadside clump of chicory for the return of her faithless lover and eventually died, her heart broken by disappointment. Chicory's long tap root digs deep into the soil and is very hard to pull out, but it is a sensitive plant in other ways. When the flowers are picked, and so separated from the plant, they lose colour and dry out almost at once.

Accepting Chicory as a core remedy is both a relief and a gift. A relief because it sheds light on darkness and enables me to accept parts of myself I might prefer to deny. And a gift because the remedies are only there to help. If I notice any unhelpful Chicory characteristics surfacing I have the power to take positive action. I can choose to heal if I am sufficiently aware and remember to act. – Kate Anderson

beatles and milligan

In the early 1970s I loved pop music, and the Beatles in particular. They were splitting up and made the news a lot, so there were plenty of chances to feed my obsession. I remember listening to a Sunday evening radio series that told their history from the Cavern Club on. I saved my pocket money for weeks to buy a greatest hits LP from the record stall in the North End Road market. I wrote my own bouncy songs, making them sound as much as possible like 'She Loves You' and 'Can't Buy Me Love'. I haunted a local department store one Christmas when they put a large yellow submarine in their toy department. I was always ready to argue, passionately and with complete conviction, that the Beatles were the greatest group there ever had been and – more unreasonably – ever would be.

When I was eleven I moved to secondary school. In one craft lesson the teacher told us we would make a paperweight using clear resin in the next class. We had to bring something in with us to put in the resin before it set. Because of my obsession I decided at once that my paperweight had to have a Beatles theme. The only thing I had that was small enough to fit in the paper cup mould was a Beatles medallion. It wasn't a real one – just a picture cut out of a *Blue Peter* annual with some irrelevant text about something or other on the other side. So I used that. Classmates poured resin over flowers, metal men, cogs and watch-springs and other interesting three-dimensional shapes. They produced interesting and beautiful paperweights. I ended up with a rather sad and pointless little thing.

Over-enthusiasm does this. It leads us to shut down parts of our life and turn away from new and unexpected possibilities in order to give all our energies to one area. We achieve more in one direction than our less focused friends – I probably knew more Beatles lyrics than most kids my age – but only at a cost. We miss more and sometimes more important things, the side turnings that less focused people wander down, some of them leading to better routes.

At its most extreme over-enthusiasm shades into a kind of mad perfectionism. The great comic writer Spike Milligan experienced manic periods during which he wrote up to fourteen hours a day, driven on by his need to be better than anybody else at comedy. During *The Goon Show* years he would write one half-hour show a week for twenty-six weeks out of every fifty-two. This would be tough going for a team of writers, but Milligan worked alone. Later similar bursts of energy accompanied him into the writing of books. Once he wrote 10,000 words in a single day, unable to stop or control what he was doing. 'I was pressured inside,' he said. 'All I could think of was the book.' In this kind of manic state people's creative output can rise significantly for a time. But without self-control and the ability to pace oneself the output can't be sustained. For manic-depressives like Milligan there is the fall from being ten feet off the ground into the depths of depression; for over-enthusiasts and workaholics generally there is exhaustion and burn-out.

see the other side: vervain

Ambassadors in the ancient world used to carry *Verbena officinalis* to demonstrate their defiance and – after a fight – their willingness to reach an understanding. And Pliny said that sprinkling vervain-steeped water around a dining room was a sure way to make guests get on with each other. The flower essence Vervain echoes these traditions. It relates to flexibility and openness. It lets us enjoy our pastimes and feel passionate about them without losing our sense of perspective. It helps us balance periods of intense work with time for rest and play. We can switch off and reflect so as to reach understanding, rather than running forever on the treadmill.

Whether supporting her favourite pop group, campaigning for the rights of political prisoners, selling soap powder or collecting money for flood relief the Vervain needs to believe in what she does and needs to see it as the right and just thing to do. As balance is lost she forgets that other people's values might be different and loses her ability to understand contradictory arguments and points of view. Her desire to discuss and persuade and win hearts and minds warps into a determination to convert others at all costs. She becomes fanatical about whatever cause she is championing and refuses to let go or give in. The Vervain campaigner becomes the terrorist; a passion for justice leads to unjust acts. Her energy and enthusiasm, from being delightful and invigorating to those around her, become a fire that burns all it touches. She can't stop or rest or distract herself. Even if she falls ill she will continue to throw herself into her work, long after most people would have retired to bed, with the inevitable consequences for her long-term health. If she has no alternative but to stop her energy will gnaw away at her so that she becomes nervous, frustrated and restless. And at a lower level of imbalance, like me with my ugly paperweight, she allows her enthusiasm for one thing to swamp other values and considerations, closing off avenues instead of opening them up.

Enthusiasm is an attractive thing. It is interested and committed and full of life. Even out-of-balance enthusiasm – absolute conviction with an endless capacity for work and activity around one compressed area – is valued and rewarded by our out-of-balance culture. And there is always something admirable in the true Vervain's commitment to the wider community. Negative Vervain people are usually happy to think of themselves as Vervains, then, and may even refuse to take the remedy because they *want* to stay active all the time – they like it that way. This is always their choice, but it misses the fact that *being* is as important as *doing*. Taking the flower allows us to let go and take time to *be*. This is Vervain's lesson.

As a child I would throw myself into tasks such as polishing shoes. I have receding gums from brushing my teeth too vigorously. I was also a perfectionist in my work. When typing I would clench my teeth and type as fast as possible. I ended up with repetitive strain injury – now greatly relieved by homoeopathy and of course increased self-awareness through Vervain. – Alice Walkingshaw

My first selection of remedies included Vervain. I didn't notice any great difference, but my family did. Apparently I became a lot easier to live with, not being as forthright as I usually was about various subjects that came up, and a lot more open with my emotions. I didn't realise these changes for quite a while, even though my family told me about them. – Jeff Chambers

In my enthusiasm for the remedies I began experimenting on a daily basis with how I was feeling and what I could take for it. It was new and great fun but a bit intense – I was desperately trying to identify new negative states. I took Vervain to lessen my zeal! – Karen Briscombe

value difference: beech

I believe a leaf of grass is no less than the journey-work of the stars,
And the pismire is equally perfect, and a grain of sand, and the
egg of the wren,
And the tree toad is a chef-d'oeuvre for the highest,
And the running blackberry would adorn the parlors of heaven.

– Walt Whitman, *Leaves of Grass*

People have long thought of beech as a holy tree that gives protection and comfort. If we pray under a beech tree the tree will send our prayer straight to heaven. If we sleep under a beech tree we will be protected from harm. We can make a sweet-smelling mattress using dried beech leaves and their rustling will whisper softly to us as we sleep. But beeches require high standards. They stand proud of the forest floor on their high roots. If we blaspheme under a beech tree the leaves will whisper against us and according to legend the tree may drop a branch on our head as a rebuke.

In a negative Beech state we are rather too ready to drop branches on those we don't agree with. If Vervain is a disciple who wants to convert, negative Beech is an Old Testament prophet with fire and brimstone ready to hand. 'I know what's right,' she says. 'If you see things differently you must be too stupid to see what is obviously true.' A mild Beech state has us criticising or making snide remarks about our neighbour's way of dressing or the kind of music our parents or children prefer. A more extreme state sees us condemn outright the habits, activities, even the existence of others. Negative Beech is the snob who despises poor and ill-educated people because they are poor and ill-educated, and never stops to think how her own wealth and privilege are the result of accident more than merit. It is the colonialist, seeking to export his view of life and progress to other cultures and unable to see that their ways might be right for them. It is the xenophobe, irritated and angered by other ways of life and seeking to place high walls around her own so as to 'protect' it, and the racist, unable to tolerate those with different coloured skin. It is the worst kind of missionary evangelist, the one who can make no allowances for difference nor understand why others might see the world and God differently.

A negative Beech attitude is hard on other people, but it hurts the Beech person just as much. If we always look for the faults in others we lose the ability to see truth and goodness. First our neighbours seem stupid, then our family, our hobbies, our goals, nature itself. Instead of expanding our souls we shrink them to a tight band of fixed and correct ideas. Instead of aspiring to the divine position of saying 'yes' to the world we end up saying 'no' to its endless and beautiful possibilities. Taking the Beech remedy helps us overcome our prejudices. It gives us the humility to accept instead of condemning. 'It is obvious that none of us is in a position to judge or criticise,' says Bach, 'for the wisest of us sees and knows only the minutest fragment of the great scheme of all things, and we cannot judge, knowing so little, how the great plan will work.' Positive Beech doesn't expect everyone to be the same. She knows there are many paths to growth and that each is valid in its own way. She seeks out the goodness in others and encourages the good that is in them. By accepting others she develops her own soul. She is more able to see the patterns in life and to appreciate them even if they violate her principles; and she has the flexibility to change her principles when she has outgrown them. This too is a form of growth.

Looking back on various unhappy episodes I realise that virtually all the problems I had with people in the past have been caused by my feeling critical of them and their various habits. Now, three months later, I can see the positive side of people who once drove me to distraction and have lost my fear of falling out with them. I no longer feel that my emotions are in charge of me. – Caroline

When I am to be involved in a meeting with people whose views I find difficult I use Beech to help me be more tolerant. It has made a big difference in the way I react. – Alison

Beech was one of the remedies I was certain I would never need. I saw myself as fair, tolerant and easy-going. But as my self-awareness developed I started hearing those little voices of criticism aimed at others. Although I always tried to appear pleasant I found that secretly I was quite judgemental and intolerant – a painful but growthful revelation. I now find that Beech helps me to see the good in others and accept them for who they are. – Michael Hillier

guide others: vine

The Vine person knows what should be done for the best. She is confident, ambitious and sure of herself, and always prepared to take command of situations and of other people. As these qualities fall out of balance, however, a darker side begins to emerge. The Vine person begins to expect obedience and make demands where she ought to make requests. She begins to feel that she knows better than anybody else, and her certainty justifies her in forcing others to do things her way. She will use her strength of character to overrule objections or turn to aggression and threats. At the most negative extreme she becomes a tyrant, yanking at the reins of her family, her employees, even whole communities so that cruelty steers them her way. She will not stop to consider the negative effect this has on other people. She is not concerned with getting affection, like Chicory, or with winning people over to her ideas, like Vervain. She just wants obedience.

The negative Vine state is full of power. But power of this kind snares and deludes us. We are trapped as surely as our victim. This is what Bach meant when he called our victims our enemies:

> In our heart of hearts we must know that our enemies are those who give way to us, because by so doing they make a bond, a bond we find almost impossible to break and we thank them when they struggle free.
>
> Anyone over whom we can influence our will or control or power is a danger to our freedom. No matter whether our influence is due to love or power or fear or what they get from us. Our souls must thank all those who refuse to be our servants, since it robs them and us of our individuality.

As with the Chicory state, too much rule over others leads us away from our destiny and stops us from growing into ourselves. And the behaviour of *Vitis vinifera* echoes the existential dilemma of the out-of-balance Vine person. It is a wonderfully rampant plant, quickly outstripping others and forcing its way through the densest growth. Yet at the same time it is tied to other plants. Although it looks dominant it is in fact a sort of parasite. It strangles the plants it climbs through. It relies on their weakness for its height instead of relying on its own strength.

The positive qualities of the Vine flower are related to understanding and wisdom. The Vine person keeps her assurance and confidence, but instead of using her gifts to control other people and force them her way she tries to guide others into their own paths – paths that will be different from her own. Instead of a tyrant she is a teacher who builds confidence and self-awareness in herself and in others. She understands that many paths can lead to many goals, all of them valuable, including those that she personally would not choose.

the philosophy of pleasure

The Greek philosopher Epicurus was born in 341 BC in Samos. He studied with various teachers and lived in Athens for a time before beginning his teaching career at Mitylene and Lampsacus. After five years he returned to Athens, where he became known for a new philosophy that taught that pleasure was good. 'The beginning and root of every good thing is the pleasure of the belly,' he wrote, and elsewhere added,

> 'I don't know how I shall conceive of the good if I take away the pleasures of taste, if I take away sexual pleasure, if I take away the pleasure of hearing, and if I take away the sweet emotions that are caused by the sight of beautiful forms.'

With the backing of wealthy friends and supporters Epicurus founded schools all around the Mediterranean, from Syria to Gaul, from Judea to Italy. They were co-educational establishments at a time when most schools were for men only, a fact that encouraged the scurrilous gossip that started to circulate about Epicurus' profligate lifestyle. He was said to over-eat so much that he was obliged to vomit twice a day. Erotic letters were published in his name, supposedly written while he was drunk. His enemies called him uneducated, promiscuous, an enemy of reason and thought, gluttonous and irredeemably vulgar, a man concerned only with the body and with a hole where the spirit should be. Even today, as Alain de Botton points out in *The Consolations of Philosophy*, those ancient rumours find an echo in the way his name is used in the names of lifestyle magazines and high-class restaurants. The fat man gorging on truffles and caviar, the spoilt playboy picking up debutantes at a casino, the pop star snorting cocaine, the movie actress drinking champagne by the pool: these dedicated consumers are the modern Epicureans.

Epicurus then and now is done a disservice by this caricature. 'The pleasant life,' he said, 'is produced, not by a string of drinking bouts and revelries, nor by the enjoyment of boys and women, nor by fish and the other items on an expensive menu, but by sober reasoning.' Epicurus defined pleasure as a simple, virtuous life in harmony with nature. The true Epicurean 'revels in the pleasures of the body on a diet of bread and water'. As he said, 'it is not possible to live pleasurably without living sensibly and nobly and justly.' Real pleasure is a quiet conscience, friends, a place to sleep, good food, and a good life: all the values that downshifters espouse today. True to these principles Epicurus lived in a shared house and enjoyed simple meals. He took part in the communal gardening that brought food to the table. His usual drink was plain water.

Epicurus was a victim of words. His use of the word 'pleasure' blinded his fellow citizens to the essentials of his philosophy. Then as now humanity assumed an opposition between 'pleasure' and 'simplicity', between enjoyment and spirituality, between physical satisfaction and goodness, so that having one rules out having the other. Epicurus says this is wrong. A good dinner and a good soul go together. Certainly Bach – who enjoyed a few pints of beer and a sing-song in the pub – wouldn't disagree. 'Life does not demand of us unthinkable sacrifice,' he wrote. 'It asks us to travel its journey with joy in our heart and to be a blessing to those around, so that if we leave the world just that trifle better for our visit, then have we done our work.'

free your soul: rock water

Even committed smokers see giving up smoking as a worthwhile goal. When we are over the craving pleasure increases in so many areas – from the smell of clean hands to the taste of kisses – that few would accuse the ex-addict of needlessly denying herself an honest, harmless pleasure, or of wearing a hair-shirt for the sake of it. What do we think, however, of those people whose good resolutions take more extreme turns? Is there a remedy to help the already healthy person who decides to give up her morning tea on principle? Or the rapier-thin woman who will never under any circumstances eat a single piece of the cocoa-rich chocolate that she and her body crave?

Often people in this state look first at the same essences as the new-born and struggling ex-smoker: Walnut to cast off the evil influence of the pleasure; Centaury to help say 'no' to the pleasure; Crab Apple to cleanse their bodies of dirty desire for the pleasure; Chestnut Bud to stop them falling once more into a state of sin by consuming the pleasure. This is unfortunate, because it looks for an answer in the wrong direction. Like the man who once marched into the consulting room at the Bach Centre and told John Ramsell without room for argument that he needed all thirty-eight remedies except Vine, the last flower people in this frame of mind will select will be the one they need: Rock Water.

Rock Water has a special place in this book, and there is no accident in its being the last remedy in *Bloom* (and the last in Bach's own *The Twelve Healers*). All through this book we have seen how the negative state often grows out of too much of the positive: Centaury helpers turn to slaves, Vine guides turn to tyrants. In the Rock Water state the subject of this book, personal growth, grows out of proportion and turns into the distortion of martyrdom. This is a state of spiritual pride, and Bach had some interesting things to say on this subject. 'In main principal,' he wrote, the fault on earth is the desire for worldly things, but the greater danger is the greed and too great desire for spiritual things. The desire to be good, the desire to be God, may be as great a hindrance in spiritual life as the desire for gold or power is in earthly experience.

Concentrating too much on our spiritual development narrows the focus of our consciousness and of our lives. We no longer see at the edges. We miss the true insight and understanding that our intuition would offer us if only we would relax and let go.

For those who are already on the path to self-realisation this is doubly important. 'The further one advances the greater must be the humility and the patience and the desire to serve,' Bach says. 'It is the state of being, not aspiring, the being brings its own reward. There must be no desire for rapid improvement or perfection, but to wait humbly content in any station or service until called to a higher. The way is impersonal service not for the sake of gaining spiritual promotion but just for the desire to serve.' The warning here is clear: if we try to go too fast and rise above 'common' humanity we are almost certainly allowing our self-interested ego to take over. We are not perfect selves, so any selfish drive for perfection will also be imperfect and take us in the wrong direction.

We need Rock Water when we make a spiritual guide out of our ego. We don't allow ourselves a piece of chocolate or a cup of tea because it would be a fall from grace. We become strict and unforgiving towards ourselves and take a hard pleasure from denying ourselves joy. We give up more and more things and construct more and more rules and prohibitions in the (sometimes unexpressed) hope that perfection will follow the final renunciation: today chocolate, tomorrow the mortal world of sin and death. We want to be an example to others and use our rigorous downshifting to demonstrate how advanced we are. Yet we are not openly critical of other people's failings because our own perfection is what matters to us above all else. There is a discord in the out-of-balance Rock Water person: a display of superiority on the outside while inside all is repression and punishment. I am never good enough for me, we say, but I can still be an example to *them*.

Rock Water states happen when we forget that the main aim of life is not to achieve the smooth perfection of a superhuman, but to be who we are. Balance comes when our personalities can flourish in the way that is right for them and in the way that does most good to our spiritual selves. Rock Water is a living symbol of balance, combining the hard (yang) and the soft (yin) in one image. Jesus built his church upon the rock Peter (in Latin, *Petra*, meaning rock) and Jesus himself is called the Rock of Ages, the foundation of all things. Rock is a positive symbol of strength and determination and irrevocable decision, and at the same time a negative metaphor for hardness and an inability to compromise. Water by contrast seems weak and inconstant. Yet water erodes the rock and reshapes it, for as the ancient Chinese philosopher Laozi pointed out, the softest thing overcomes the hardest. The tide smooths jagged stone to still pebbles and the stream clefts the hardest earth to find its path.

To find the best way forward in our spiritual development we need to balance the rock and the water, the yang and the yin: stand firm, but remain fluid, stick to our beliefs and principles, but still show flexibility and softness to our blossoming selves. The Rock Water remedy reminds us that the true way of growth is upwards and outwards: expression, not repression. It allows the essential part of us to guide growth in a natural way, taking directions and forms that we can never find with our conscious minds alone. It helps us turn away from the hard fight of the pilgrim and instead find truth in the quiet meadows, among the birds and flowers. In Bach's words these drops are 'the pure springs gushing from the rocks, bringing brightness and refreshment to those weary and sore after battle'.

I always wanted to learn to swim but fear of water stopped me. Every week I put myself through misery trying to learn but couldn't seem to overcome the fear despite taking Rescue™ Remedy and Mimulus. It wasn't until I recognised the Rock Water trait in myself – setting myself impossible targets each week which I could never hope to reach, instead of being satisfied with slow progress, that I began to get anywhere.
– Chris

One morning I found myself staring into the mirror, tidying my appearance and preparing for the day. To my horror, I heard myself say, quite sharply and bossily, 'Come on, hurry up, you haven't got time for this!' I suddenly realised that I had been doing this sort of thing for years, and had never wanted to look at it consciously. I turned back to the mirror and said, 'It's all right, you don't need to talk to me like that.' I started working with Rock Water. It helped me to reach a more comfortable and peaceful internal relationship. – Michael Hillier

My personal life is hugely supported by the remedies. Over the last seven months, since treating myself as a Rock Water type, I have found that I have become rounder, softer and more forgiving of myself. – Elaine Copeland

I caught myself in the supermarket one day holding a box of pure vegetable soap in such a way that I hoped a passing shopper would see what it was. I viewed my sister's visits as an opportunity to let her see what she should be eating – I used to eat only good wholesome food, no cakes, pastry or chocolate biscuits. I can laugh about it now. – Alice Walkingshaw

directions

I was learning to drive. I was a nervous learner because I was so conscious of the danger inherent in driving. This small white hatchback was a half-ton lethal weapon. So as I drove along the streets I looked at all the things I was desperate not to hit. The car followed where my eyes led, and I seemed to be forever veering towards and steering away from pedestrians, cyclists, other cars, bollards and kerbstones. Eventually my instructor gave me some good advice. 'Don't look where you don't want to go,' he said, 'look where you want to get to.'

This advice applies to more than steering cars down Fulham Palace Road. We magnify whatever we turn our attention towards. For example:

❀ In *Lessons from the Art of Juggling* Michael Gelb and Tony Buzan tell the story of a golfer who drove a ball into a particular water trap four times in a row during a golf championship. When he came back the following year he assured journalists that he had solved the problem because he had given it so much thought. But when he got to the same hole he swung and – inevitably – put the ball straight into the water again.

❀ When Robert Holden, the founder of the Happiness Project, was training to be a psychologist his training concentrated on the many forms of schizophrenia, depression and anxiety. At the end of a week studying depression all the psychology class was depressed. At no time did anybody suggest that these future healers of the mind should look at happiness, contentment and spiritual growth. So when Holden started his career he expected to find psychological disorders (and consequently found them) in everybody who came to see him.

We can all think of similar examples from our own lives. If we go into a job interview thinking about all the wrong things we shouldn't say the chances are we will say the wrong things. Cigarettes will rule our day if we think too much about the need not to smoke. Concentrate on not drinking and at once the TV and the high street are full of invitations to go back on the booze. But if we think about the ways we can get things right, about strengths and positive experiences and outcomes, then those are the things we magnify. We open up possibilities and make success easier than failure. By looking at the cyclists and oncoming buses and all the other things I didn't want to hit I made them larger and harder to avoid. Once I switched my focus to the gaps between the bikes and the buses, the gaps got bigger and I sailed through.

This is why Bach recommended that we should not take the Rock Water route and fight against our failings. Fighting against them is a way of concentrating on them and making them bigger. It strengthens the very negative it is supposed to suppress. 'Hate may be conquered by a greater hate,' said Bach, 'but it can only be cured by love: cruelty may be prevented by a greater cruelty, but only eliminated when the qualities of sympathy and pity have developed: one fear may be lost and forgotten in the presence of a greater fear, but the real cure of all fear is perfect courage.' Trying to repress a negative feeling using force or cruelty or condemnation doesn't remove the poison. The negative remains boxed inside us and festers, always threatening to break out again when we are weak or tired. Like an alcoholic thinking about not drinking, we see the incipient negative in everything we do. It colours every waking moment. The only healthy thing to do with an unhealthy emotion is to cultivate the high and healthy so that we can literally feel better: 'in spiritual advancement,' said Bach, 'we must always seek good to drive out evil, love to conquer hate, and light to dispel darkness.'

Edward Bach's thirty-eight healers don't swamp or override or battle against our negative feelings. They don't mask or repress, like some hippie version of Prozac. Instead they transform. They turn our minds to what is good in us, to our qualities, and to the qualities that we want to develop. The negative stuff gets smaller once we look beyond it. Or, as my driving instructor could have said, 'Don't think about what you don't want to be, think about what you can be.' When we do this we see at once how big our inner potential is. There's plenty of room in there to bloom.

appendix 1
❧ summary

I sometimes finish reading a book and think, Well, what was that all about? In case you're thinking that now, here is a summary of *Bloom*'s structure and argument.

structure

As you will remember from the introduction, this book was structured something like a labyrinth. There were three main 'paths'.

❧ In the first path (chapters 1 to 7) I looked at personal and spiritual development and at how the thirty-eight remedies relate to downshifting, peak and plateau experiences and different schools of religious and philosophical belief. I also used this space to make a political argument about how we should best use essences.

❧ The second (chapters i to vii) covered the individual remedies in the system and said when to take each flower and what it would do for us.

❧ The third path was a combination of the first two: the two sets of chapters were interleaved so that you could read both in the order in which they arrived.

The diagram shows the main theme or themes in each chapter. The arrows show the three main reading schemes you could have used; there are of course many other alternative paths you could pick back and forth through the labyrinth.

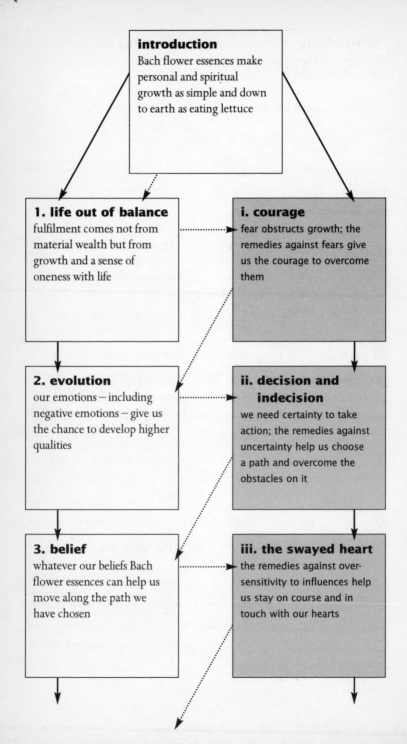

introduction
Bach flower essences make personal and spiritual growth as simple and down to earth as eating lettuce

1. life out of balance
fulfilment comes not from material wealth but from growth and a sense of oneness with life

i. courage
fear obstructs growth; the remedies against fears give us the courage to overcome them

2. evolution
our emotions – including negative emotions – give us the chance to develop higher qualities

ii. decision and indecision
we need certainty to take action; the remedies against uncertainty help us choose a path and overcome the obstacles on it

3. belief
whatever our beliefs Bach flower essences can help us move along the path we have chosen

iii. the swayed heart
the remedies against over-sensitivity to influences help us stay on course and in touch with our hearts

4. simplicity

Bach stripped away inessentials; his system of thirty-eight essences balances simplicity and effectiveness

iv. living today

to advance we have to be present in the moment; the remedies against insufficient interest help us focus and act

5. peaks and paradigms

at the highest points of insight people see the universe as a simple whole; flower essences and simple methods are natural stepping stones towards insight

v. connecting

the three remedies against loneliness help us connect with others and with the world

6. towards intuition

moving closer to our feelings moves us closer to our souls; taking essences in the simplest way we learn from our lives and move towards perfect intuition

vi. positivity

the remedies against despondency and despair help us find the positive in every situation, even when all hope seems gone

7. steps along the path

the simple way of using remedies builds on the wisdom of the labyrinth, that sees value in the slow and winding journey of self-discovery

vii. give freedom, get freedom

our path is our own; others have other paths to walk; we should not seek to control others, or ourselves, but walk our path with patience and humility

the argument

The motif of the labyrinth was a key element in *Bloom*. The book swirled back and forth around this and other themes so that mazes, paths, simplicity, speed and stillness came up and came back over and over. This echoed the central message of the book, which was that flower essences represent a slow and organic way of growth that involves understanding emotions and experiences and then revisiting them, each time with more insight. Patience and slowness are necessary for genuine growth. Forced self-cultivation is like using chemical fertilisers on the soil: it gets quick results but scars the earth. Genuine long-term growth means the slow overcoming of our negative states, so that the ways in which we choose to work with Bach flower remedies will dictate the quality of the results we achieve. I believe and hope you will have got most from this book if you read through the third path and followed every line of the argument; the two short cuts inevitably meant missing out on things, as short cuts often do.

✺ using the system

the moment of crisis

Most people don't start using the remedies out of a desire for personal growth. Instead almost everybody starts with the most famous of the remedies, the ready-prepared mix best known under the trade name Rescue™ Remedy. The story told by Helen, a schoolteacher from the north of England, is typical of the thousands of first contacts that take place every week somewhere in the world.

> My first experience of the remedies was one evening six years ago when I scalded myself in the steam of a pan. I was already feeling very wound up and unhappy, and I burst into tears. The unopened Rescue™ Remedy was sitting on the kitchen shelf and I decided to try it. I sprinkled it all over my burning forearm and took several drops on my tongue. The effect was dramatic and entirely unexpected. Within seconds I experienced a feeling of deep peace. All the unhappiness and tension I'd been feeling melted away. I went to bed and slept for twelve hours, and when I woke up I felt completely rested and still with this lovely feeling of peacefulness. There was a tiny patch of blistering on my arm which I had missed from covering with Rescue™ Remedy, otherwise my skin was unaffected.

Obviously, serious burns would require professional medical treatment, but even in the case of a real medical emergency Rescue™ Remedy can help keep us calm and focused. It contains Star of Bethlehem for recovery from shock, Impatiens to calm general agitation and the rushed feeling caused by too much adrenaline, Cherry Plum to help us keep our self-control, Rock Rose to calm panic and Clematis to keep us grounded and aware of our surroundings. This formula was laid down by Dr Bach, who put the combination together as a first-aid measure for situations in which there wasn't time to sit down and think about a careful selection of remedies.

There are three main reasons for Rescue™ Remedy 's overwhelming popularity among first-time users.

✿ **It is the only remedy whose use is clearly indicated by its name**. At the time of writing legal restrictions on the labelling of complementary medicines mean that flower essence makers can't always say on the bottle what their remedies do. Someone who wanders into a pharmacy looking for something to keep him calm during a job interview has no way of knowing that Mimulus deals with fear, Larch with lack of confidence and so on, but it's clear that the situation is an emergency of sorts so a rescuing remedy must be a good choice.

✿ **It is the only one that doesn't require introspection**. All the single remedies treat very specific emotional states, the idea being that you select one or several to match the way you feel. Doing this requires some measure of self-analysis, and in today's quick-fix over-the-counter culture many prefer the pre-prepared option.

✿ **It is very good at doing what it says on the bottle**. Rescue™ Remedy really does help calm our jangled nerves in emergencies and get us through sticky situations.

Because of these advantages some of us never move beyond Rescue™ Remedy. We shelter under it month after month through a succession of emotional storms, never stopping to ask why our lives are so full of wind and wuthering. One student wrote: 'The first remedy I used was Rescue™ Remedy. I liked the name. Well, I thought, I have taken that remedy so everything will be OK now. I treated it as a panacea and didn't look up what was in it for quite some time. When I did it didn't really mean much to me as I was quite out of touch emotionally.'

Like taking an aspirin against toothache, daily use of Rescue™ Remedy may kill the pain and help us carry on but it won't address the real problem. To do this we need to look beyond the crisis and select the single remedies that will help us deal with its cause. Instead of Rescue™ Remedy *alone*, we should think Rescue™ Remedy *and then* or Rescue™ Remedy *plus*. This is what Sandra, another teacher, did at a particularly bad time in her life:

> I was desperate, thought I would try them but was not expect-
> ing anything from them, prioritised my concerns and bought a
> bottle of Rescue™ Remedy plus a selection for my panic attacks.
> I told no one. After three weeks I felt ordinary and normal –
> nothing special or spectacular, just ordinary and calm. I found
> I was able to distance myself from work at home and that
> difficult children at school didn't drain or upset me as they used
> to. Someone I worked with and knew very well remarked on it.
> Until her remarks I hadn't noticed anything dramatic or revolu-
> tionary. The whole process was totally imperceptible.

simple uses

From one angle Bach remedies are a complementary system of medicine like any other. Their special strength is helping with emotional and behavioural problems like depression, agoraphobia and chronic stress. But we can also use them when we are physically ill, usually as a back-up to other therapies. If we have irritable bowel syndrome or asthma or any other stress-related disorder we use them to help manage stress. If we have cancer we use them to help us cope with the rigours of orthodox cancer treatments such as chemotherapy and surgery. Feeling happier in ourselves helps us cope better with our physical symptoms. It also helps our immune systems function better, and our bodies will be better able to return to their own natural state of health.

From another angle Bach remedies are a simple means of self-help. 'When I feel out of balance I reach for the remedies and feel their vibrations melt away my negativity like snow in the sunshine,' says one Australian remedy user. 'They bring me back to my centre again.' So if we feel tired at the end of a long day we put two drops of Olive into a glass of water to help restore our energy levels. If we can't stop worrying over something that happened at work we take White Chestnut. If we are anxious about giving a speech we take Mimulus, or Larch if we are sure we will make a mess of it because we are no good at that kind of thing. This was the kind of use that Nora Weeks remembered Edward Bach talking about: 'I want to make it as simple as this: I am hungry, I will go and pull a lettuce from the garden for my tea; I am frightened and ill, I will take a dose of Mimulus.'

When I first started I only used the remedies when I was desperate, like I would use painkillers. As I've grown with them they have become part of my life. I'm constantly learning more about them. They help me even before I have swallowed them, as they encourage me to open up to myself and really look at how and what I am feeling. I am more in touch with my body and with my emotions and thoughts. – Judy Beveridge

I found the immediate effect quite subtle but nevertheless there was a definite change. I felt in contact with a higher vibration within myself, bathed in a gentle energy, more centred, more calm. I was intrigued. – Richard

Learning about the remedies has been like finding the key to a door I always wanted to walk through. I think Bach all the time now. – Pamela Wells

deeper uses, just as simple

'It seems that my use of the remedies deals with two sides of me,' says Bach practitioner Christine Racquez. 'The first addresses passing moods that are easy to recognise if I stop to look and am honest with myself. The second is linked with personal growth and is much more difficult to deal with because it concerns my whole self since its beginnings.'

From this third angle immediate self-help graduates into personal development. Having dealt with our tiredness at the end of every working day we begin to look at and address the reasons we are tired. We might think about the things we want to change. Perhaps we want to give up smoking or find a different job or be less impatient with our family or build more fulfilling relationships with our lovers and friends. We see how the essences can help us break out of negative patterns and find ways forward. And there is a fourth angle that relates to our ultimate spiritual development. What do we want to do with our lives? How can we find meaning and a sense of purpose? What are we here for? The essences won't provide off-the-peg answers to these questions, but they can help us work out a way to find our own individual made-to-measure solutions.

The third and fourth ways of using essences go hand in hand, just as personal and spiritual development do. We need to define and make meaningful changes on a personal level if we want to get to where we can go spiritually, for there is no point having a goal if we don't make changes towards it. And personal changes only have meaning if we can see how they work towards something, for there is no point making change for the sake of change. Spiritual and personal development are two faces of a single coin.

> At first I used them infrequently and usually when there was a sense of dissatisfaction with my life – a need to know why I was feeling as I did. Sometimes I felt I was searching for something within myself and the remedies would spring to mind. I felt they were teaching me about myself. – Elaine

I look deeper and notice how I react and respond to different situations, people and things. The remedies connect me to earth, to spirit, to other people and to myself. They help me know myself and others on a deeper level. I have been able to love and accept parts of myself that I would not have even recognised before. They help me to develop and change. They have been invaluable. – Judy Beveridge

acceptance

'Initially it made me feel worse about myself when I read some of the remedy descriptions,' says Alison, who started using Bach essences in 1990 when she became a foster carer. 'I would see myself as this dreadful person experiencing these awful emotions. I remember putting off using one or two such as Beech and Holly as I felt I would be admitting I was this horrible, intolerant, vengeful person.'

Most books on Bach's work concentrate on describing negative emotions. They do this for excellent reasons, because we need to know what negative emotions a flower treats if we are going to know when to select it. But we have seen how thinking in negatives brings risks and can lead us to overlook the positive. We must never do this, not when looking at the essences and not when looking in our own hearts. As Bach himself pointed out in 1930, the negatives are always and only a means to an end: 'we only judge the faults and failings and the adverse circumstances of a patient as indications of the good he is endeavouring to develop.'

We sometimes forget this and get into the habit of condemning ourselves for the way we feel. If we feel angry about something our first thought is that we are wrong to feel like that. If we are afraid of something that is a *stupid* thing to feel. If we feel despondent we *lose patience* with ourselves at once. This is one way that onions build up. The original feeling gets buried until we lose sight of what it was, but the pain of it remains along with the self-condemnation it generated, both unresolved and growing and feeding each other. To break the circle we need to put self-condemnation aside and accept our emotions for what they are: not part of us, and so not an occasion for self-condemnation, but something that we feel, something that will pass, something that we can overcome. Acceptance is the first step. It really is OK to feel angry or afraid or despondent – everybody feels that way sometimes. 'My use of the flowers has resulted in my being able to be more honest with myself,' says Bach practitioner Margaret Blackman. 'I can acknowledge that "nasty" feelings are human and common to us all at times.' The next step, just as important, is to learn from our feelings and use them to move towards the positive, as Margaret has done. 'Choosing a remedy whilst in a negative emotional state has enabled me to move on in my own personal growth path with the result that life is much calmer and richer.' Anger is a chance to learn love, fear a chance to learn courage, despondency a chance to learn joy. Negative emotions are welcome once we can accept and name them and look at them in the right way.

Change requires some letting go and a new insight. Just thinking in terms of the remedies helps me to let go. They have done more for me in two and a half years than twenty-five years of self-examination and struggle and running away ever did.
– Charles Callis

keeping a journal

'I have a notebook in which I've recorded every batch of remedies I've mixed myself since 1992,' says Angela Davies, a practitioner who teaches about Bach's work in the UK and Switzerland. She isn't alone. Keeping a journal is encouraged on Bach Foundation-approved courses as a good way of charting growth and learning more about who we are. It gives us a chance to record our feelings and thoughts and experiences taking essences. How did we feel when we took that remedy? What quality did we aim to strengthen? And what did we actually achieve?

As well as dealing with the day-to-day reality of getting in touch with our feelings, a remedy journal is a good place to ask basic questions about our lives. What have we learned from this experience, that emotion, this remedy? How will we do things differently next time? How far were other people helping or harming us? Have we set our personal boundaries to give us space to do what we need to do? Are we really being who we are, expressing our higher self through our every action and thought?

Given the nature of these questions we will probably keep our remedy journal private most of the time. This is our space in which to explore and accept ourselves; and sometimes writing a journal helps uncover a whole new layer of imbalance that needs addressing. This is what Angela found. 'When I first started taking remedies regularly I included Impatiens and Holly,' she says. 'Within a month the headaches I had suffered with regularly for ten years disappeared completely. I rejoiced at my good fortune in discovering the remedies when all other self-help methods had failed, but as I continued I began to discover much fear underneath the anger. This is something I am continuing to work with.' This degree of self-awareness and self-acceptance is the only genuine road to self-improvement, because it means working with what's there rather than pumping up our egos with dreams and fantasies.

There are many ways to write a remedy journal. We can treat it as an autobiography or a novel. We can lay it out as a table, with the left-hand side dedicated to what was actually happening (where we were, who else was there, what we were doing), the middle detailing how we felt and the right-hand side listing the essences we took and the results we got. Or we can use short cryptic notes or non-linear methods like mind-mapping or drawing. Any method that works is fine.

selecting and taking

Most people take flower essences by mouth, which is discreet, effective, quick and convenient. You can dilute them before you take them or take two drops at a time neat from the bottle you buy in the shops. (In the jargon, the remedies in the shops are stock bottles. A 20ml stock bottle contains 1.3 drops of active mother tincture.) Whether you dilute the stock remedies or not makes no difference to the way they work, but if you don't dilute them you will take in more alcohol, use up more essences and spend more money.

There are two ways of taking diluted remedies. For immediate use add two drops of each selected stock remedy to a glass of water. It doesn't matter how much water is in the glass. It doesn't make any difference if you add more drops. Then sip as often as you need to. You can mix up to seven remedies together at one time. If you put a lot of different essences in you are probably including some you don't need, which tends to obscure the effect of the ones you do need. Keep it simple and only select what you are sure you need.

If you want to take the remedies over a longer period of time it is more convenient to make up a mix in a bottle that you can carry around with you. Mixed bottles are known as *treatment bottles* or *personal dosage bottles*.

To make up a treatment bottle put two drops of each selected remedy into an empty 30 ml (1 oz) glass bottle. Use the kind with a dropper built into the cap if possible. If you can't get this exact size bottle any smaller size will do. Top the bottle up with non-fizzy mineral water. You could add a teaspoon of brandy or cider vinegar first if you want to, as this helps keep the water fresh. The dosage from a mixed bottle is four drops taken at regular intervals, and at least four times a day. If you haven't added a preservative keep the bottle in a cool place – the refrigerator is fine. Avoid storing any remedies in direct sunlight, as this reduces their shelf-life.

If you want to take Rescue™ Remedy remember that the dosage is four drops from the stock bottle, not two. So you could take four drops neat in your mouth in an emergency or add four drops to your glass of water or treatment bottle. If you are mixing Rescue™ Remedy with other remedies the Rescue counts as a single remedy. In other words you can add Rescue™ Remedy and up to six other remedies to your mix.

Flower essences are very safe and can be used alongside most other types of treatment and medication. There are no contraindications to flower essences themselves – i.e. the energised water that is made using the sun or boiling method. But they are bottled in alcohol, one of the commonest and most natural of preservatives, which is used as a carrying medium and to keep the mother tincture fresh. Bach used to allow chemists to use rectified spirits when he supplied them with mother tinctures, but his own preference was for brandy because it was a natural product. This is why the Bach Centre and its commercial partners still use brandy in the mother tinctures, stock bottles and pre-pared treatment bottles. If you are especially sensitive to alcohol for any reason you will want to seek the advice of a qualified medical adviser before you take them. To get the alcohol problem in perspective, if you use the treatment bottle method and don't add extra brandy to the bottle you will only be taking two or three drops of alcohol over a period of up to three weeks. For most purposes this amount of alcohol can be disregarded.

The glass of water and treatment bottle mixes are the classic ways of taking essences. But you can use them in other ways if you want to. They are far more robust than homoeopathic medicines, so you can add them (neat or diluted) to fruit juice, tea, coffee and other drinks, or even take them in food if you prefer. Many people like to add their drops to their bath water or use plant sprayers to mist the room with favourite essences. People with a religious or medical objection to alcohol may be able to use them externally, applying the drops to pulse points at the wrists, temples and neck.

things that don't matter

Most medicines come with a long list of don'ts: don't drink, don't drive, don't take on a full or empty stomach and so on. Taking Bach essences is different. The only don'ts are the ones we saw in the previous section. Rather than a long list of don'ts, then, here is a list of things that don't matter.

❀ The size of the glass of water. Just take bigger sips.

❀ Taking remedies through x-ray machines or keeping them next to the microwave oven. Neither will affect the essences.

❀ Keeping remedies in the refrigerator. This won't affect the essences.

❀ Keeping remedies near aromatherapy oils etc. Won't affect the essences.

❀ When you last ate. Makes no difference to the effect.

❀ Taking the remedies every few seconds. Isn't dangerous.

❀ Taking remedies for years at a time. Isn't habit-forming.

❀ Adding vodka or vinegar or whisky to your treatment bottle as a preservative instead of brandy. No problem. Brandy isn't an active ingredient.

❀ Taking them when you are pregnant. Won't hurt you or your baby.

❀ Using tap water instead of mineral water. Won't keep fresh as long, but the remedies work the same.

❀ Using fizzy mineral water in a treatment bottle. Will run over the side of the bottle as it fizzes up, but the remedies work the same.

❀ Putting more than two drops in a treatment bottle. The remedies work just the same.

❀ Putting the water in the treatment bottle before putting the drops in. Makes no difference.

✿ Forgetting to take remedies. Is often a sign that you don't need them any more, or that you aren't ready to make a change yet.

✿ Taking them neat instead of diluted. Makes no difference to the effect.

✿ Taking them diluted instead of neat. Makes no difference to the effect.

✿ Taking them without professional advice. Is never dangerous.

✿ Taking the wrong remedies. Won't help you, but won't make things worse.

Many of these questions come up again and again, often because authors who should know better have mentioned them as areas of concern. Bach essences are safe, kind, gentle and positive. They are perfect for self-help. We just need to take what we need when we need it. If we are anxious and worried about taking them we should start with Mimulus, or Aspen, or White Chestnut.

essence checklist

Agrimony – mental torture behind a cheerful face – see page 68

Aspen – fear of unknown things – see page 19

Beech – intolerance – see page 204

Centaury – the inability to say 'no' – see page 71

Cerato – lack of trust in one's own decisions – see page 44

Cherry Plum – fear of the mind giving way – see page 22

Chestnut Bud – failure to learn from mistakes – see page 109

Chicory – selfish, possessive love – see page 199

Clematis – dreaming of the future without working in the present – see page 110

Crab Apple – the cleansing remedy – see page 165

Elm – overwhelmed by responsibility – see page 173

Gentian – discouragement after a setback – see page 49

Gorse – hopelessness and despair – see page 50

Heather – self-centredness and self-concern – see page 140

Holly – hatred, envy and jealousy – see page 80

Honeysuckle – living in the past – see page 104

Hornbeam – procrastination, tiredness at the thought of doing something
    – see page 46

Impatiens – impatience – see page 133

Larch – lack of confidence – see page 176

Mimulus – fear of known things – see page 17

Mustard – deep gloom for no reason – see page 113

Oak – the plodder who keeps going past the point of exhaustion –
    see page 172

Olive – exhaustion following mental or physical effort – see page 105

Pine – guilt – see page 177

Red Chestnut – over-concern for the welfare of loved ones – see page 24

Rock Rose – terror and fright – see page 19

Rock Water – self-denial, rigidity and self-repression – see page 210

Scleranthus – inability to choose between alternatives – see page 42

Star of Bethlehem – shock – see page 163

Sweet Chestnut – extreme anguish, the dark night of the soul – see page 161

Vervain – over-enthusiasm – see page 202

Vine – dominance – see page 206

Walnut – protection from change and unwanted influences – see page 76

Water Violet – reserved pride and aloofness – see page 137

White Chestnut – unwanted thoughts and mental arguments – see page 99

Wild Oat – uncertainty over one's direction in life – see page 39

Wild Rose – drifting, resignation, apathy – see page 103

Willow – self-pity and resentment – see page 168

appendix 3
✻ learning more

the bach centre

The best-known brand of Bach flower essences – look for the signature on the bottle – contains mother tinctures made at Mount Vernon, the Oxfordshire cottage where Edward Bach spent the last years of his life. The Bach Centre provides free help and information on Bach and his work and a mail order service for books. The house and gardens (which are owned by a charitable Trust) are open to the public.

Formed in 1991 to oversee the Bach Centre's educational work, the Dr Edward Bach Foundation runs or approves courses in more than twenty countries around the world. The Foundation's International Register of Practitioners lists over 1,500 trained practitioners who work using Dr Bach's simple and open approach to health. The letters BFRP after a practitioner's name indicates that he or she is registered with the Foundation. The Foundation operates a strict Code of Practice and can refer callers to local practitioners.

> The Dr Edward Bach Centre
> Mount Vernon
> Bakers Lane
> Sotwell
> Oxon OX10 0PZ
> UK
> Tel: 00 44 (0) 1491 834678
> Fax: 00 44 (0) 1491 825022
> www.bachcentre.com
> mail@bachcentre.com

further reading

Assagioli, Roberto, *Psychosynthesis*, Viking Press, 1973

Attali, Jacques, *Chemins de sagesse*, Fayard, 1996

Bach, Edward, *Heal Thyself*, CW Daniel Co, 1931

Bach, Edward, *The Twelve Healers and Other Remedies*, CW Daniel Co, 1936

Baker, Margaret, *Discovering the Folklore of Plants*, Shire Publications, 1999

Ball, Stefan, *Bach Flower Remedies for Men*, CW Daniel Co, 1996

Ball, Stefan, *The Bach Remedies Workbook*, CW Daniel Co, 1998

Ball, Stefan, *Principles of Bach Flower Remedies*, Thorsons, 1999

Ball, Stefan, *Teach Yourself Bach Flower Remedies*, Hodder & Stoughton, 2000

Bloom, William (ed.), *The New Age*, Rider, 1991

Boardman, John et al., *The Oxford History of the Classical World*, Oxford University Press, 1986

Bono, Edward de, *Simplicity*, Viking Books, 1998

Botton, Alain de, *The Consolations of Philosophy*, Hamish Hamilton, 2000

Brockman, John and Matson, Katinka (eds.), *How Things Are*, Weidenfeld & Nicolson, 1995

Camus, Albert, *Le mythe de Sisyphe*, Gallimard, 1942

Camus, Albert, *Carnets, janvier 1942 – mars 1951*, Gallimard, 1964

Capra, Fritjof, *The Tao of Physics*, Flamingo, 1989

Chancellor, Philip, *Illustrated Handbook of the Bach Flower Remedies*, CW Daniel Co, revised edition, 1990.

Claxton, Guy, *Hare Brain Tortoise Mind*, Fourth Estate, 1997

Durning, Alan Thein, *How Much is Enough? - The Consumer Society and the Future of the Earth*, W.W. Norton & Co, 1992

Eliot, T.S., *Collected Poems 1909–1962*, Faber and Faber, 1963

Ferguson, Marilyn, *The Aquarian Conspiracy*, Paladin Books, 1982

Gelb, Michael and Buzan, Tony, *Lessons from the Art of Juggling*, Aurum Press, 1995

Gleick, James, *Chaos*, William Heinemann, 1988

Goleman, Daniel, *Emotional Intelligence*, Bloomsbury Publishing, 1996

Goodall, Jane, *Reason for Hope*, Thorsons, 1999

Handy, Charles, *The Hungry Spirit*, Hutchinson, 1997

Hesse, Hermann, *Steppenwolf*, Penguin Books, 1965

Holden, Robert, *Happiness Now!*, Hodder & Stoughton, 1998

Kotre, John, *White Gloves: How We Create Ourselves Through Memory*, Free Press, 1995

Kuhn, Thomas, *The Structure of Scientific Revolutions*, University of Chicago Press, 2nd edition, 1970

Lapham, Lewis H., *Money and Class in America: Notes and Observations on Our Civil Religion*, Weidenfeld & Nicolson, 1988

Levi, Primo, *If this is a Man/The Truce*, Penguin Books, 1979

Lovelock, James, *Gaia – A New Look at Life on Earth*, Oxford University Press, 1982

Mackenzie, Donald, *Myths and Legends: China and Japan*, Studio Editions, 1986

Martin, Paul, *The Sickening Mind*, HarperCollins, 1997

Maslow, Abraham, *Religions, Values, and Peak Experiences*, Penguin Arkana, 1994

Maslow, Abraham, *Towards a Psychology of Being*, John Wiley and Sons, 1998

McGreal, Ian (ed.), *Great Thinkers of the Eastern World*, HarperCollins, 1995

McGuire Thompson, Gerry, *Encyclopedia of the New Age*, Time Life Books, 1999

Meyer, Tom, *Powers of the Soul*, Laser Pages Publishing, 2000

Milligan, Spike and Clare, Anthony, *Depression and How to Survive It*, Ebury Press, 1993

Myers, David, *The Pursuit of Happiness*, Avon Books, 1993

Ramsell, John, *Questions & Answers: the Bach Flower Remedies*, CW Daniel Co, revised edition, 1996

Ramsell, John and Ramsell Howard, Judy (eds.), *The Original Writings of Edward Bach*, CW Daniel Co, 1990

Ramsell Howard, Judy, *Bach Flower Remedies Step by Step*, Vermilion, 2005

Ramsell Howard, Judy, *Bach Flower Remedies for Women*, Vermilion, 2005

Ramsell Howard, Judy, *Growing Up with Bach Flower Remedies*, CW Daniel Co, 1994

Scheffer, Mechthild, *Bach Flower Therapy*, Thorsons, 1990

Spaemann, Robert, *Notions fondamentales de morale*, Flammarion, 1999

Spark, Muriel, *The Prime of Miss Jean Brodie*, Macmillan, 1961

Stapledon, Olaf, *Last and First Men*, Millennium, 1999

Thoreau, Henry, *Walden*, Oxford University Press, 1999

Veenhoven, Ruut, 'Advances In Understanding Happiness', *Revue Québécoise de Psychologie*, vol. 18, 1997

Weeks, Nora, *The Medical Discoveries of Edward Bach, Physician*, CW Daniel Co, 1940

Weeks, Nora and Bullen, Victor, *Bach Flower Remedies: Illustrations and Preparations*, CW Daniel Co, 1964

Whyte, David, *The Heart Aroused*, Industrial Society, 1997

Wilson, Colin, *The Outsider*, Victor Gollancz, 1956

✿ index